Professional and Therapeutic Boundaries in Forensic Mental Health Practice

Forensic Focus

This series, edited by Gwen Adshead, takes the field of Forensic Psychotherapy as its focal point, offering a forum for the presentation of theoretical and clinical issues. It embraces such influential neighbouring disciplines as language, law, literature, criminology, ethics and philosophy, as well as psychiatry and psychology, its established progenitors. Gwen Adshead is Consultant Forensic Psychotherapist and Lecturer in Forensic Psychotherapy at Broadmoor Hospital.

other titles in this series

Therapeutic Relationships with Offenders
An Introduction to the Psychodynamics of Forensic Mental Health Nursing
Edited by Anne Aiyegbusi and Jenifer Clarke-Moore
ISBN 978 1 84310 949 5
eISBN 978 1 84642 890 6

Personality Disorder
The Definitive Reader
Edited by Gwen Adshead and Caroline Jacob
ISBN 978 1 84310 640 1
eISBN 978 1 84642 864 7

Forensic Issues in Adolescents with Developmental Disabilities
Edited by Ernest Gralton
ISBN 978 1 84905 144 6
eISBN 978 0 85700 346 1

Psychiatry in Prisons
A Comprehensive Handbook
Edited by Simon Wilson and Ian Cumming
ISBN 978 1 84310 223 6
eISBN 978 0 85700 206 8

Sexual Offending and Mental Health
Multidisciplinary Management in the Community
Edited by Julia Houston and Sarah Galloway
ISBN 978 1 84310 550 3
eISBN 978 1 84642 785 5

Forensic Focus 35

Professional and Therapeutic Boundaries in Forensic Mental Health Practice

Edited by Anne Aiyegbusi and Gillian Kelly

Jessica Kingsley *Publishers*
London and Philadelphia

First published in 2012
by Jessica Kingsley Publishers
116 Pentonville Road
London N1 9JB, UK
and
400 Market Street, Suite 400
Philadelphia, PA 19106, USA

www.jkp.com

Library of Congress Cataloging in Publication Data
Professional and therapeutic boundaries in forensic mental health practice / edited by Anne Aiyegbusi and Gillian Kelly.
  p. ; cm.
Includes bibliographical references and index.
ISBN 978-1-84905-139-2 (alk. paper)
I. Aiyegbusi, Anne. II. Kelly, Gillian, 1978-
[DNLM: 1. Forensic Psychiatry--ethics. 2. Professional-Patient Relations. W 740]

  614.15--dc23
                          2012005077

British Library Cataloguing in Publication Data
A CIP catalogue record for this book is available from the British Library

ISBN 978 1 84905 139 2
eISBN 978 0 85700 328 7

Printed and bound in Great Britain

CONTENTS

INTRODUCTION

People who become detained in or use forensic mental health services are defined by the fact they have violated boundaries, often in multiple ways. Societal laws, organisational rules, other people's bodies and/or other people's lives are included in the toll of destruction which in turn is often a re-enactment of violations they have suffered. For clinicians employed to work therapeutically with this client group, the capacity to initiate and maintain boundaries is critical to safety as well as good treatment outcomes. This, however, sometimes occurs in the midst of an immense onslaught of pressure to seriously transgress and operate outside of the professional role.

Such experiences may be apparent during interpersonal relations with patients or, less obviously, in relationships with colleagues where the interpersonal dramas of the patient group may be graphically mirrored. A further possibility is that the clinician does not experience themselves to be either in violation of their professional role or on the slippery slope towards such a situation. Indeed, the clinician may feel themselves to be 'called upon' as only they can provide curative interventions for a particular patient. Likewise, clinicians may feel themselves to be powerfully in love with the patient and not question this.

As unpalatable as some of these suggestions are, most forensic clinicians will have encountered similar scenarios during their working lives. An unfortunate characteristic of clinical scenarios involving boundary violations by professionals, especially sexual boundary violations, is that the patient may be viewed as the perpetrator rather than the victim, especially if the patient is male and personality disordered, and the staff member is female. This may be a reflection of how complex and interrelated the picture is, in terms of vulnerability and risk, while also highlighting the fact that some gender issues in forensic settings may simply not be fully understood.

This book sets out to address the challenges of working in a boundaried way within forensic services from numerous perspectives. The authors are highly experienced practitioners in forensic and related fields who share their perspectives on boundary implications for working with people who have experienced profound victimisation and/or have offended significantly. A range of treatment settings are included, from community outpatient clinics to high security hospitals.

In Chapter 1, **Gwen Adshead** locates professional boundaries in the context of ethics, arguing that boundary violations represent a failure of ethical reasoning. In exploring the reasons why boundary violations may be more common in forensic practice, it is suggested that there are features of forensic work that are so disturbing that professionals 'can turn a blind eye' to what is happening in front of them.

The next two chapters address phenomena of victims and perpetrators of boundary violations in mental health work, especially psychological therapies. In Chapter 2, **Dawn Devereux** offers a much-needed, predominately UK perspective on the patient's experience of professional abuse in the psychological therapies. In reviewing existing literature on the subject, the reader's attention is brought sharply to the considerable iatrogenic harm caused by these encounters with professionals who violate treatment boundaries. In Chapter 3 by **Jonathan Coe and Glen Gabbard**, Jonathan Coe skilfully conducts an interview with Professor Gabbard, the aim of which is to explore issues surrounding the risk and rehabilitation potentials of professionals who have violated professional boundaries with patients. The chapter offers unique insights into the experience and expertise of Professor Gabbard at The Gabbard Center, an international centre of expertise in Houston, Texas. Numerous issues are discussed, including the approach to assessing individuals' potential for risk and rehabilitation, post-rehabilitation monitoring arrangements, victim issues, types of transgressor, risk factors, epidemiology, denial, cultural influences and much more.

The next series of chapters explore treatment modalities for boundary-violating patients. In Chapter 4, **David Jones** considers sexual offending, its relationship to healthy sexuality, the cultural and legal slipperiness of such terms and the nature of criminality encompassing such extreme boundary violations. Light is shed on the complex and challenging implications for psychotherapeutic work with men who have offended sexually, with the risks to the therapist of being drawn into a perverse therapeutic relationship clearly described. In Chapter 5, **Estelle Moore and Emma Ramsden** write about the power of a therapeutic group approach for men who have offended, are receiving treatment in a high security psychiatric hospital and who have a history of boundary violations while detained. The devastating consequences of abuse of interpersonal boundaries, its multiple intergenerational impacts via connection to further offending and its implications for those detained are acknowledged. This chapter raises awareness of the challenges such men may struggle with some understanding of why they may have engaged in severe boundary violations in custodial settings. In Chapter 6, **Mario Guarnieri** explores boundary phenomena in forensic dramatherapy, drawing upon his experiences within the dramatherapy space to highlight creative ways of working with a patient's verbal and non-verbal expressions of internal boundary confusion. The significance of and interplay between both a boundaried space and the experience of a boundaried therapeutic relationship are discussed. The clinical example is used to bring depth to the discussions and elucidate the multiple boundary issues that arise and can be explored as well as worked through in forensic dramatherapy. In Chapter 7, **Stella Compton Dickinson and Andy Benn** have focused on boundary phenomena in the practice of forensic music therapy for patients receiving treatment in secure hospital settings. Various boundary issues which are important to pay attention to, such as confidentiality and security procedures, are discussed in the context of the secure treatment environment, followed by an explanation of how the intra-psychic world of the forensic patient may become apparent through musical expressions, which may also be jointly created with the therapist. In Chapter 8, **Jo Bownas** introduces aspects of working with boundaries in family therapy in a secure inpatient setting. The chapter is constructed around a clinical vignette which brings the clinical work to life, providing the reader with insight into some of the theories, practices and intentions of family therapy approaches to working with boundaries in the forensic setting.

The next three chapters focus on forensic mental health nursing, providing different perspectives on the nursing task with people who transgress boundaries. In Chapter 9, **Gillian Kelly and Emma Wadey** explore boundary phenomena from a nursing perspective. The chapter highlights how the very nature of forensic nursing can bring about complex boundary issues and how these issues can be compounded by numerous systemic factors. Consideration is given to the requirements of nurses working in forensic settings as well as the importance of fostering organisational cultures that are proactive and progressive in their responses not only to boundary transgressions but also to the needs of nursing staff and patients in relation to the maintenance of professional and therapeutic boundaries. The development of a boundaries workshop is also discussed. In Chapter 10, **Cindy Peternelj-Taylor** addresses issues of boundaries and desire in forensic mental health nursing. The scope and potential scale of sexual boundary violations as well as factors that influence sexual boundary violations from a nursing perspective are explored. The management of risk in relation to boundaries is considered, paying particular attention to individual, peer and organisational responsibilities. Areas for practice and research development in this field are usefully discussed. Then in Chapter 11, **Anne Aiyegbusi** describes boundary phenomena and boundary violations in the nurse–patient relationship with people diagnosed with personality disorders in a high security psychiatric hospital Dangerous and Severe Personality Disorder (DSPD) service for men and a Women's Enhanced Medium Secure Service (WEMSS). The clinical experience of nurses and patients is presented through findings that emerged from a mixed methods research study. This study highlights the interpersonal pressure applied to nurses to operate outside of their professional role in these services where risk and vulnerability are so tightly intertwined. Also, it is suggested that a key nursing task is to withstand this pressure as part of the overall multi-disciplinary treatment task of supporting patients to discontinue destructive patterns of relating.

Some different treatment settings are considered in the following three chapters. In Chapter 12, **Brian Darnley, David Reiss and Gabriel Kirtchuk** explore some of the boundary challenges inherent in forensic settings. Using psychodynamic theory and clinical example the authors discuss the complex interplay of dynamics that can occur between staff and patients and ultimately lead to the re-enactment of a patient's early life experiences with concomitant boundary violations. The chapter discusses how the development of an Interpersonal Dynamics tool and meetings support clinicians in understanding patients, including the dynamics of boundary phenomena that can repeatedly occur with patients. In Chapter 13, **Claire Dimond and Denise Sullivan** explore boundaries within an adolescent forensic unit. The authors consider what constitutes safe and developmentally appropriate boundaries. They draw on legal and clinical frameworks as well as refer to contexts in which boundaries have been violated in the form of child abuse. Theoretical and clinical approaches that inform the authors' practice in managing boundaries within an adolescent unit are also discussed. In Chapter 14, **Rebecca Neeld and Tom Clarke** explore boundaries and the nurse–patient relationship within the context of a therapeutic community. The role of containing boundaries in fostering mentalisation with people diagnosed with personality disorders is explored. Importantly, the subtle process of utilising boundary crossings on the part of the nurse to foster reparation within the therapeutic relationship is extremely well presented through a clinical example.

Particular diagnoses and clinical phenomena associated with boundary violations are considered in the next four chapters. In Chapter 15, **Kingsley Norton** explores boundaries and borderline personality disorder. Boundaries in relation to professional and patient roles are considered, including the impact of the characteristics of borderline personality disorder on both the patients' abilities to maintain boundaries as well as the abilities of the professionals caring for them. The importance of boundary crossings in terms of providing valuable clinical information and as indicators of more harmful boundary transgressions are highlighted. Dynamics of care and control are explored, as are the impact of interpersonal stressors emanating from internal and external sources. Monitoring the boundaries of role is discussed, including the use of inference in this process. The importance of professionals reflecting, both individually and in teams, on their roles in relation to patients' needs and the wider forensic setting, be it inpatient or community, are emphasised. The value of patients being supported to know and understand acceptable boundary behaviours is also discussed. In Chapter 16, **Derek Perkins** describes professional and therapeutic boundaries from the perspective of working with men who have seriously offended and who have been diagnosed with severe personality disorders. Models of personality disorder and psychopathy are described, along with considerations for treatment and management in clinical and custodial settings. The role of maintaining safe boundaries with this group of men is placed in the context of risk management and treatment requirements. The characteristics of severe personality disorder that manifest in boundary-violating scenarios are thoroughly explored. In Chapter 17, **Anna Motz** explores three different types of boundary failures in maternal care and the serious harm these cause. The first is one where the mother cannot see the baby as a separate person; the second is found within a toxic partnership in which each partner projects significant aspects of themselves into the other and disowns them. Self-harm is the third manifestation of boundary failure described in this chapter. Case examples are employed and, as a result, these complex processes are made clear to the reader. In Chapter 18, **Richard Curen** begins by raising the long-standing debate about the institutional care of people with learning disabilities and, in particular, those described as having 'challenging behaviour'. Reference is made to recent media coverage of abuse of learning disabled people in residential care. The overwhelming experiences of rejection, abandonment, trauma and hatred that learning disabled people may live with on a day-to-day basis are clarified along with the learning disabled offender's defence against this pain which may involve victimising others. Concepts such as 'the disability transference' and 'secondary disability' are brought to life through riveting case examples.

In Chapter 19, **Christopher Scanlon and John Adlam** describe Bentham's panopticon: a design for a form of an eighteenth-century correctional facility in which the living quarters of the inmates would be sufficiently transparent that they could be viewed from all angles at any time by unseen attendants. It is proposed that the parallel fear observed in staff working in secure settings in the present day can be considered in terms of an anxious perversion of the dynamic of the panopticon. In Chapter 20, **Stephen Mackie** writes about his experience of when the boundary in a psychiatric ward staff team is not specific and delineated but appears to be avoided or absent and develops into a hidden protective space. The author discusses this boundary phenomenon in relation to a reflective practice group and highlights how the use of boundary as a defence inhibits its usefulness as a protected containing space. Finally, in Chapter 21, **Ronald Doctor and Maggie McAlister** explain how homicide is the ultimate boundary violation. This chapter explores how such acts may be understood and also how professionals can be aware of re-enactments in therapeutic relationships. The psychopathology of homicide, considering how clinicians might work effectively and safely with the homicidal patient, is considered in this chapter.

Chapter 1

WHAT THE EYE DOESN'T SEE: RELATIONSHIPS, BOUNDARIES AND FORENSIC MENTAL HEALTH

Gwen Adshead[1]

Overview

Boundary violations represent a failure of ethical reasoning by professionals. In this chapter I explore the reasons why boundary violations may be more common in forensic practice by examining models of caring relationships in mental health care, and the particular demands of forensic mental health. Specifically, I will argue that there are features of forensic mental health care that are so disturbing that professionals can turn a 'blind eye' to what is happening in front of them. There is therefore a compelling need for supervision and clinical oversight of all therapeutic relationships in long-stay residential psychiatric care, especially in forensic settings.

INTRODUCTION

A boundary defines a space with an inside and an outside. The contents of one space do not go into another space. The professional boundary not only defines

---

1   This chapter draws on expert testimony given to the Kerr Haslam Inquiry in 2004 and work with Jonathan Coe at the Clinic for Boundaries Studies (previously Witness), a charity providing support for people abused by professionals); and evaluation and education of boundary-violating professionals. However, the views in this paper are entirely my own and do not represent the views of other professionals nor those who employ me. I have chosen to use the term 'professional' because all professionals can be involved in boundary violations. Similarly, I have also chosen to use the term 'patients'.

the identity of the professional, it also helps to keep personal and professional identities apart. Keeping the boundary involves the way one speaks, what one wears, how one acts and other non-verbal and unconscious interactions.

Boundary violations occur when elements from the personal space intrude into the professional space and to some extent, vice versa. Sarkar (2004) suggests that boundary-violating health care professionals are struggling with the 'who-ness' and 'what-ness' of their work, where the professional identity is the 'what-ness' of a person, and the personal is the 'who-ness'. If the who-ness of a person gets too confused with the what-ness, there may be a loss of professional identity and disturbance of the therapeutic relationship.

Anecdotally and empirically, we know that therapeutic relationships are harmed when professionals cross boundaries in terms of harm to the therapeutic alliance and work, harm to patients directly, and harm to services as a whole. In forensic residential settings, such boundary violations may significantly impair security for everyone.

Models of care-giving relationships and ethics

All relationships can be defined in terms of the time spent together, the depth of the connection and the mutuality between the parties (Cox 1988). Traditionally, health care relationships may involve varying amounts of time together, and they may also vary in their depth, in terms of degrees of intimacy. In terms of mutuality, health care relationships frequently entail real inequalities of power and vulnerability because people seeking care are usually in a vulnerable and dependent condition when they seek help. Vulnerable and dependent people can be exploited by others who are stronger and more powerful, as frequently happens in non-human primate groups (Sapolsky 2004).

These inequalities of power may be the experiential basis for the development of ethical codes in health care, where a group of people deliver care to the vulnerable and dependent. The Hippocratic corpus is one such system of thought but there are others from other ethnic and cultural traditions (Veatch 2000). What they have in common is that those with professional knowledge and well-being should not exploit those lay people who are ignorant, disabled and needy. These moral imperatives were particularly meaningful in the early history of medicine and surgery, when treatments were physically hazardous and had the potential to do more harm than good: hence the imperative, 'Do no harm'.

As medicine and nursing developed as formal professions, with bodies of specialist knowledge and skills, so too did conceptual models of professional relationships in health care (see Box 1.1). First, and most traditional, is the *parental* model of health care whereby the professional acts in a parental role, as the wise adult who combines specialist knowledge with caring for vulnerable patients rendered powerless by their condition. The professional's primary duty is to protect the patient from harm (including distress) and try to promote the patient's welfare. The patient's autonomy is secondary to his/her well-being, which is defined by the professional and not the patient.

BOX 1.1 MODELS OF HEALTH RELATIONSHIPS (VEATCH 1972)

Models of relationships in health care

- Parental/priestly
- Engineer or technician
- Contractual/fiduciary
- Collegial
- Advocate/covenant

Such a model places the patient in a child-like role because of their vulnerability and need for protection. They are passive, while health care professionals are active. The parental model may be perfectly appropriate for people who are very ill, and who lack capacity to exercise their own autonomy because of their disease or disorder. However, the parental model will be inappropriate for patients who still retain capacity to be autonomous or who are disabled, not disordered or where the clinical problem is one of fluctuating autonomy. In mental health, the patient's problem is one of fluctuating autonomy, or living with a disabling condition. They may or may not lack capacity to make decisions for themselves (Okai *et al.* 2007). Overriding a competent person's wishes is deemed to be authoritarian or paternalistic (Szasz 1989), especially in mental health, where the enhancement and restoration of autonomy is a key clinical activity.

There are three other models of health care relationships that have currency in health care systems. They are the engineering model, the contractual model and the collegial model. In the *engineering* model, the health care professional is a technical expert, and the body is seen as a machine to be 'fixed'. The professional presents the facts about treatment to the patient without making any value judgements, and the patient makes the final decision. The professional provides a 'service' and the patient is therefore a 'service user'.

Under the *contractual* model, there are obligations and benefits for both parties. Though their interests may not be identical, the parameters of the relationship allow for the interests of both to be achieved to a reasonable extent. The patient is a client and the professional is a provider. If either party decides that they cannot continue with the relationship due to disagreement or conscience, then the contract is either broken or not made in the first place. Both parties maintain a degree of control and individuality. Such a model may be formalised in legal terms as a signed contract with financial penalties if either side defaults. This is obviously the model that applies in private health care settings; and in public health it is best applied to elective interventions with people who have full capacity and are not in great distress or discomfort.

A more nuanced version of contractual relationships are *fiduciary* relationships, which are based on trust, loyalty and truthfulness and which then give rise to legal obligations; for example, a fiduciary relationship may be the basis for a legal Trust. In health care, fiduciary relationships are contractual in the sense that there is a relationship of trust in which the patient counts on the health care provider to both care for and care about a patient as a person. Such an approach may be utilised with people who have less capacity or autonomy on a temporary basis.

Finally, the *collegial* model sees patient and professional as colleagues attempting to pursue a common goal. They treat each other as equals, and have trust and confidence in each other. Both are respected for contributing important pieces of information in an effort to agree on a specific treatment plan. Patients are referred to as patients and their autonomy is shared with the clinical team, who have their best interests at heart. The recovery approach in mental health has something in common with the collegial model, whereby there is a recognition of the skills and experience that both parties bring (Frese *et al.* 2001).

Veatch (1972) is describing models largely based on *medical* relationships with patients. However, it is often argued that nurses have qualitatively different experiences and views of the relationship. For example, Bernal (1992) describes an advocacy model of nurse–patient relationships which is both contextual and holistic. As an advocate for the patient, the nurse not only protects but promotes the patient's rights and interests; perhaps even taking up a position against the more parental model of the doctor. Bernal also describes a *covenant* model in which the nurse 'covenants' with society to provide the best service he can, based on his professional knowledge and skills. The covenant model sees the nurse cooperating with a group of people to provide care, as opposed to the advocacy model that does not consider third party interests.

There is no space to critique these models in detail here. The key point is that each model describes a different kind of relationship between the patient and the professional. Another key point is that each model varies in the balance of power and autonomy between the parties. Finally, the different models each give rise to different frameworks for understanding professional ethics and duties. In the parental model, the clinician has a duty of care to protect the vulnerable patient's welfare and that takes precedence over other duties. In the collegial model, the duty is to respect the patient's (or client's) growth and well-being by having respect for their personal autonomy.

These different ethical frameworks give rise to different models of professional communication and behaviours. For example, a nurse or doctor who sees the therapeutic relationship as a purely technical or contractual one will communicate and interact with the patient in a different way to the professional who sees the patient as a 'child' to be protected. This can in certain circumstances lead to disputes between professionals about how best to treat patients (Main 1957).

The nature of care-giving relationships in mental health care

By definition, to be mentally unwell is to have one's autonomy impaired to some degree and for some period of time. People with psychiatric disorders are made uniquely vulnerable by their disorders. Not only do they suffer distress, but their capacity to regulate feelings, make judgements and protect themselves can be impaired. It is therefore crucial for patients to be able to feel that they can trust the professionals who care for them at their most vulnerable. In addition, psychiatric patients are vulnerable because in most Anglo-European countries, the state has legislation that gives mental health care professionals powers to detain people who seem to be mentally unwell and whose disorder leads them to pose a risk to themselves or others. Some countries even give professionals power to prescribe and administer treatment in the absence of consent or in the face of a flat refusal. There are thus real power disparities between psychiatric patients and professionals that could be exploited by either party.

If we look at Veatch's (1972, 2000) models of health care relationships, it seems unlikely that models demanding high levels of autonomy will meet patients' needs when they are at their most distressed and disorganised. However, many patients will be able to move to a different type of relationship, given time and help. Mental health professionals therefore need skill in being able to 'read' the relationship, and respond flexibly, sometimes being parental, sometimes contractual, sometimes collegial, and always open, communicative and transparent.

The parental model of mental health care is still dominant in psychiatry and is often criticised for being patronising and disrespectful. Although there is much truth in this criticism, what it does not address is the fact that patients may need to be vulnerable and child-like at certain times, and for that vulnerability and neediness to be respected and cared for, without abuse. Health care culture has changed over the last 40 years and now rightly promotes patient choice, autonomy and control over their disorders, but it is also vital that health care cultures respect human vulnerability and frailty. Studies of the attachment bonds in mammals show that it is natural (and inevitable) that when we feel sick and unwell, we often want someone to 'take care' of us, and that being 'taken care of' leads to recovery of strength and independence (Bowlby 1970). The attachment literature also reminds us that patients' own attachment histories will have a profound effect on how they seek care from professionals and how they engage in and work with treatment (Henderson 1974; Dozier *et al.* 2001).

Attachment issues are likely to be particularly problematic in mental health because the majority of service users will have insecure attachment histories and styles, which impact on how they relate to psychiatric professionals (Adshead 1998; van IJzendoorn and Bakermans Kranenburg 2008). There is evidence that patient attachment style has an influence on both the development of the therapeutic alliance and compliance with therapeutic regimes (Dozier *et al.* 2001). Patients from insecure backgrounds may find it hard to be patient, grateful or compliant or may be reluctant to take responsibility for themselves when they feel vulnerable. Those who have had unbounderied relationships with previous care-givers may assume that lack of boundaries is the norm in any relationship where there are disparities of knowledge or experience. It may be hard to stick to a collegial relationship with a patient if they act 'as if' you are a seductive or cruel parent.

Complex caring

'Taking care' of the vulnerable includes a variety of tasks, not all of which are easy. A personal and poignant description of care-giving is given by Arthur Kleinman (2009), a famous psychiatrist and anthropologist:

> [Caring] is very difficult. It is also far more complex, uncertain and unbounded than the professional medical and nursing models suggest. (p.293)

Concepts of caring are often idealised in health care and are also bound up with gender role stereotypes about femininity. But care-giving and care-eliciting may not always be easy or straightforward, especially when the care needed is long-term and does not lead to cure. Care-giving may be especially hard if the patient is difficult, hostile or mentally unwell.

Attachment theory tells us that care-eliciting and care-giving behaviours are the products of a mental conception of a caring relationship in the mind: an 'internal working model' of how to give care and receive care (Bowlby 1970, 1977). However, Veatch's (1972, 2000) accounts of health care relationships do not describe them as arising in the minds of *both* parties. Nor do these models give any hint that professionals may have feelings about their patients (beyond a kind of general compassionate detachment) or how they should manage them professionally. This is problematic for those professionals who work with patients who have highly antisocial aspects to their minds and where this antisocial aspect means that patients are derogatory about both their care and their care-givers. It is also problematic for those who work with traumatised people, who may consciously want the professional to act as type of perpetual protector, and demand special care (Main 1957). A particular challenge is working with people whose parents or carers sexualised intimacy and care, and treated the child as a sexual adult.

The bottom line is that professionals do have feelings about their patients; feelings that may be acted out in a variety of ways at work (Menzies Lyth 1988; Lowdell and Adshead 2009). Feelings may be driven by some aspect of the patient's attachment history or the professional's attachment history or (commonly) both interacting with one another. Models of health care relating that do not attend to these feelings will not help professionals to manage feelings, forcing them underground.

Sensuality, carnality and eros: caring and the body

There is not space to do justice to the role of the body in health care relationships but it seems appropriate to have some brief discussion of the issue, in the context of sexual boundary violations in particular. I have found it helpful to distinguish between different aspects of intimate physical experience: the carnal, the sensual, the sexual and the erotic (see Box 1.2). The *carnal* refers to the straightforward physical experience of flesh being touched or touching, and the tension and arousal that goes with it. The *sensual* refers to how that carnal experience is elaborated and worked on in the mind; and associated with affects, usually (but not inevitably) positive affects such as pleasure, excitement and relief from tension. The *sexual* builds on the sensual and the carnal, but is organised around the experience of a personal identity and social influences from family and culture around gender/sexual identity and role. Finally, the *erotic* entails both a coherent organisation of all of the above into a narrative of experience. This is inter-subjective and interpersonal, so that the erotic is always imbued with intentions towards another.

BOX 1.2 TYPES OF TOUCHING AND THEIR MEANING

- Carnal: no mutuality or personal engagement; may or may not be pleasurable

- Sensual: perceptual arousal, integrated with memories and other affects

- Sexual: related to personal identity, affected by family/social values about gender and sex role

- Erotic: mutual, intentional, mentalising the other, integration of sexual and sensual

---

On this account, the physical encounters of routine physical health care may be carnal and sometimes sensual. They are, however, not sexual or erotic. Nevertheless, it is not uncommon for patients to experience being touched clinically as carnal/sensual, and to respond accordingly. Many general health care professionals have had the task of managing the embarrassment of a male patient who has an erection while being bathed or catheterized.

I suggest that health care relationships cannot be erotic relationships because of the absence of mutuality in terms of both power and knowledge of the other. However, health care relationships may become *sexualised* and both parties may consent to this. One reason that health care relationships may become sexualised is that there are superficial similarities between erotic relationships between peer couples and professional caring relationships. At the most basic level, there may be exposure of the naked body in ways that are normally only associated with sexual contact or, at least, personal intimacy. In mental health, there may be personal disclosure which is also associated with emotional intimacy. In addition, for many people, the earliest memories of being cared for when distressed may be laid down as physical memories of being touched and these memories may have a sensual quality. Any kind of physical touching may stimulate unconscious memories of early touch, located in the right hippocampus, and linked to the right limbic system (Schore 1994).

Another reason that health care relationships may become sexualised is a deep wish for the erotic and intimate by either a vulnerable patient or vulnerable professional. However, if this happens, it is an abandonment of the caring role by the professional in question, and this is why it violates professional ethics.

Boundary violations in health care

It is useful to remember that the majority of boundary violations in health care relationships are *non-physical* and *non-sexual*. In general health the commonest type of boundary violation is inappropriate self-disclosure. Gossip is another common boundary violation and, in fact, the main reason for professionals being required to pay attention to confidentiality. There is concern, however, that more severe types of boundary violation start with more minor ones, like personal disclosure (Sarkar 2004).

The most egregious form of professional boundary violation is the pursuit of an emotional and sexual relationship with a patient. This has been proscribed since Hippocratic times and is probably the only health care injunction that everyone knows! Nevertheless, some doctors, nurses and psychological therapists will have been reported as being involved in such behaviour. Sexual boundary violations (SBVs) are more common in three circumstances:

1. Where there is prolonged, repeated and intimate contact between the health care provider and the patient. In general medicine, this has most commonly involved GPs, obstetricians and gynaecologists and psychiatrists or psychotherapists.

2. Where there is insecure attachment and dysfunctional care-seeking patterns by the patient. In studies of abuse by psychotherapists, the patients most at risk are those with borderline psychopathology, which is characterised by abnormal care-seeking behaviours (Main 1957). Other patients at risk are those who have previously been exploited by parental care-givers (Kluft 1990).

3. When the care provider is also struggling with attachment issues and when they do not feel cared for elsewhere, and seek care from the patient (Gabbard 1989). It is also said that there is a sub-group of professionals who are predatory and seek to exploit patient vulnerability, although how common this is in practice is hard to know.

Patients, clients and service users report being harmed by SBV. It is important to recognise that SBV is not the same as sexual assault in that there is formal consent. The wrongdoing lies in the professional allowing a relationship to change its nature from being professional to personal. Typically, the health care professional is the one who brings the relationship to an end, at which point the ex-partner/patient reports them to a disciplinary body. Clients and patients who have had sexual relationships with professional carers typically describe feeling used, betrayed, let down and distressed.

In mental health, SBV is particularly problematic because the patient or client also loses their therapist and their therapy, which they sought for personal and distressing problems, often relating to intimate relationships. SBV by mental health professionals therefore aggravates the original problem as well as causing additional distress.

The literature about SBV in health care typically describes a female patient and a male professional. Often the female patient will be particularly vulnerable in some way and the male professional will seem to offer safety and security. Both parties may justify the relationship to themselves by ceasing the therapy and finding another therapist for the patient.

Although most SBV is not a criminal offence, there are certain circumstances where criminal proceedings may follow. Under English law, it is a criminal offence for a mental health care professional to have a sexual relationship with a patient detained under the Mental Health Act in their place of work no matter how willing or consenting the patient may be.

Boundary violations in forensic mental health care (i): what do we know?

There are important differences between forensic mental health care and general mental health care, and the types and nature of professional boundary violations are also different. The starting point of analysis is the nature of the relationship between the forensic patient and the health care professional. Forensic mental health care does not easily fit any of the models in Box 1.1. Most patients will be detained under mental health legislation, and therefore experience themselves as coerced into care. Furthermore, the coercion is on the basis of prevention of harm to others so that detention is not always primarily to help the patient, but to protect the public (Eastman 1999).

Boundary violations in forensic mental health care differ from boundary violations in general mental health (see Box 1.3). In general mental health care, the commonest boundary violations are inappropriate self-disclosure and sexual boundary violations of female therapy patients by male therapists. In forensic mental health care, inappropriate self-disclosure is also common but physical and verbal abuse of patients is regularly reported. Sexual boundary violations are less common than verbal and physical abuse but usually involve female staff with male patients (Thomas-Peter and Garrett 2000). It is this author's experience that the patients are more likely to be those who are antisocial, score highly for callous and exploitative attitudes on a measure of psychopathy, and have histories of sexual offending against women.

BOX 1.3 SEXUAL BOUNDARY VIOLATIONS IN GENERAL AND FORENSIC SETTINGS BASED ON EXISTING EVIDENCE BASE

General mental health	Forensic
Female patient	Male patient
Male professional	Female professional
Patient is seeking psychological therapy or treatment	Patient is detained in hospital and may or may not be care-seeking
Patient is overtly vulnerable and may be demanding of special attention	Patient is overtly vulnerable and may be demanding of special attention OR patient may be especially charming
Patient has history of unstable relationships and childhood abuse: often sexual abuse by male protector	Patient has history of unstable relationships and childhood abuse: especially with mother, i.e. first female care-giver
Patient has no criminal history	Patient is established criminal rule-breaker
Professional may be junior or senior	Professionals tend to be senior
Professional may be under care-giving stress at home	Professional may be under care-giving stress at home
Professional may have predatory history of this behaviour	Professionals usually have good work record
Traditional health care relationship: most cases reported are in private sector	Relationship of care and control: all in state sector

There are many risk factors operating in forensic settings that increase the risk of professional boundary violations. Patient factors include:

- Seventy per cent of patients in secure settings have severe personality disorders: borderline personality disorder, antisocial personality disorder and narcissistic personality disorder. This means that they do not view interpersonal relationships in the same way as people without such disorders.

- Manipulation and deceit may be first-line interpersonal strategies for many patients, especially those who have survived extensive childhood and adult trauma.

- Previous histories of child abuse. One study of secure care found that 80 per cent of patients had experienced childhood abuse or neglect (Coid 1992). Adults who were abused as children are familiar with 'special' relationships that have a cost to them, and have to be kept secret. They may be emotionally demanding and aggressive or unusually compliant or passive with authority figures. These adults may have decreased capacities to identify threat or take action to self-protect.

- A tendency to predatory exploitation of vulnerability will be present in 25–30 per cent of patients.

- Patients are forced into a compliant and submissive role in secure settings. Some will acquiesce with this, because it is familiar from early abusive experience. Others will see themselves as unfairly abused and coerced.

- All criminal offending is a boundary violation, that is, violation of legal boundaries. Therefore forensic patients are known boundary breakers. However, they may also be in denial about their propensity to breach boundaries.

Professional risk factors can be listed as follows:

- Expectations of bringing about change by being kind and compassionate. Many forensic practitioners hope that traditional caring may bring about reduction of hostile and antisocial states of mind. It may, but it cannot be assumed. Many new practitioners are unprepared also for the degree of hostility and fear they experience from their patients.

- The degree of exposure to patients is much higher for forensic nurses than for any other health care professional. Staff in long-stay residential care will spend more hours with their patients than in personal relationships with friends and family.

- Forensic practitioners are generally not as antisocial as the patients! They are often selected for being pro-social and may react to boundary-pushing behaviour by patients with pro-social responses, which are then interpreted as vulnerability by patients.

- Fear of attack may lead to collusion and avoidance of boundary keeping. Hurt and distress in relation to fear may also generate anger and feelings of revenge.

- 'Macho' culture: how could a patient affect *me*? Staff may feel it is unprofessional, or evidence of weakness, to experience feelings about patients.

- Childhood histories of disturbed attachments in staff. Given the prevalence of childhood adversity in most populations (about 30% in most countries: Kessler *et al.* 2010), it is likely that a sub-group of forensic professionals will have histories of childhood abuse and neglect and may therefore have insecure attachment styles. In fact, attachment theory states that 'compulsive caring' is one way that people manifest insecure attachment (Bowlby 1977). This group may be vulnerable to exploitation, especially if they have some personal attachment issue going on at home, such as divorce, bereavement or family illness.

- Rates of stress and depression in forensic staff may be higher, which may increase acting out.

There are also institutional factors that contribute to an enhanced risk of boundary violations:

- Emphasis on behavioural control, not assessment of mental states or interpersonal relating.

- Formulation of the patients' problems only in terms of physical risk (e.g. hitting out), not psychological risk.

- Formulation of forensic patients as exactly like other mental health service users and 'vulnerable' in the same way.

- Denial that patients have feelings about staff and vice versa; and denial that such feelings are part of the professional challenge of residential care.

- Institutional derogation of 'talking therapies' or reflective spaces.

- Provision of 'supervision' which relates only to monitoring of tasks and targets.

- Dismissal of dissent or concerns about boundaries.

- Institutions in a state of flux and change.

- Institutions that do not learn from mistakes.

Boundary violations in forensic mental health care (ii): what do we think is going on?

The complexities of the relationships between forensic patients and professionals has long been recognised (Robinson and Kettles 1999; Aiyegbusi and Clarke-Moore 2009) and the reality of boundary violations in forensic practice has been in the public domain for over 40 years (see Box 1.4). How is it that these boundary violations continue to occur? And specifically, how do forensic professionals allow them to do so?

BOX 1.4 PUBLIC INQUIRIES IN UNPROFESSIONAL BEHAVIOUR BY FORENSIC PROFESSIONALS

1980 Inquiry into physical abuse of patients by staff at Rampton Hospital

1984 Ritchie report into death of patient at Broadmoor Hospital

1988 HAS report critical of patient care at Broadmoor Hospital

1988/89 SHSA inquiry into death of patient at Broadmoor Hospital

1991 Inquiry into the death of Orville Blackwood at Broadmoor Hospital

1992 Blom Cooper inquiry into physical abuse of patients by staff at Ashworth Hospital personality disorder unit

1999 Fallon inquiry in boundary violations by staff at Ashworth Hospital personality disorder unit

2009 NHS London inquiry into death of patient at Broadmoor Hospital (PBRL)

2010 Staff convicted of criminal offences involving SBV at Broadmoor Hospital: no public inquiry

---

There are a number of factors that may contribute to the persistence of boundary violations, described in the following sub-sections.

The limited utility of traditional models of health care relationships that are taught in training

Most professionals will enter forensic practice having assumed or been taught that one of the traditional models of health care relating is the basis for their work. It may take some time to find out that these models of care are not always helpful and professionals may lack a more complex model to guide them.

The parental model is risky in forensic services because many patients experience professionals as coercive and controlling parents who have to be managed and 'got round': a model which fits with their previous life experience. Without an internal working model of good parenting, patients often respond to kindness with confusion, hostility and fear. Contractual relationships may be possible for day-to-day matters in residential care, although the issue of sanctions for contractual infringements is complex. Overall, however, there is no contract between the patient and professionals who contain and care for them. Nor are detained patients free to make contracts in the ordinary way.

Collegial relationships imply a mutual respect for autonomy which cannot be assumed and risk management does not support. Advocacy models risk setting professionals up against other professionals on behalf of the patient in ways that cause unhelpful and fixed divisions of opinion in teams. In summary, traditional models of health care do not assist forensic professionals and there is a lack of training and support for models of care that combine compassion, self-reflection and risk management in a coherent way.

Gender and hierarchical issues

There is a real question about the extent to which disparities in power are perceived as a basis for sexual intimacy. In traditional, patriarchal societies, dominant men select less powerful women for their mates and a woman's inferior position may be taken to indicate that she is sexually available. Feminist deconstruction of power in relationships has challenged this type of power inequality as a basis for sexual congress. Nevertheless, the influence of this belief can be seen in prison settings where inferior people in the hierarchy are deemed to be sexual prey, and can be 'fucked' (literally and figuratively) if not protected. It is also no accident that sexual boundary violations in general medical care have largely been pursued by dominant men against vulnerable women, especially those who have childhood histories of being sexually 'taken' by fathers or stepfathers who saw them as (literally) 'fair game'. The metaphor from hunting is crucially accurate here.

For antisocial and predatory men, position in social hierarchies is crucial for self-esteem and masculine identity and it is reasonable to suppose that many forensic patients find it sexually humiliating to be controlled by women in positions of power. Female staff may be seen as 'fair game' by predatory patients seeking to restore their status, at least in their own minds. Of course, some patients may find it sexually arousing to be controlled by women (and men), especially those who have been exposed to sadomasochistic relationships in the past. Finally, some female staff who have been exposed to sadomasochistic relationships in their own past may find it exciting to have men (or women) under their control, or sexualise relationships with patients as a means of dealing with feelings of fear, hostility or revenge.

Compulsive repetition of dysfunctional behaviour

Freud first described this in neurosis and work based on attachment theory has confirmed the level of unconscious repetition of attachment patterns of behaviour across different relationships. In institutional settings, the repetition of offence-like behaviours with staff and other patients is called 'offence paralleling behaviours' (Daffern, Jones and Shine 2010). Although secure care may offer some physical restraint for patients' negative feelings and behaviours, acting out negative feelings may remain the first line of psychological defence for patients for many years. For sexual offenders, repetition of offending is likely to involve the most vulnerable.

What the eye doesn't see: bystanders and psychic retreats

In formal investigations into boundary violations by forensic professionals, a key question is who knew what was going on, and for how long? It is often noted that other professionals are suspicious but feel unable to act, as if they are helpless bystanders. Social psychology research from the 1970s has found that human beings are often reluctant to help those in need if others are present who could help. This reluctance to help has been called the 'bystander effect' (Latane and Darley 1970), in which people seem to absolve themselves of moral responsibility if they are part of a wider group of people also present. There is a moral question about the role of the bystander and the extent to which they 'decide' not to see what is going on because they fear others' responses or criticism. It is noteworthy that the bystander effect has *not* been studied in the caring professions, perhaps because it has been assumed that any care-giver would act when faced with an emergency situation.

It might be argued that suspicion of boundary violations does not constitute an emergency (although such violations do put security at risk) and that it is a severe accusation to make of a fellow professional. But I wonder if the bystander effect among forensic staff is generated by fear of 'seeing' something very disturbing, namely the eradication of difference between the patient and the forensic professional. John Steiner (1985) discusses how 'blind' people can be to conflicts and affects that they cannot bear to think about, and I have already referred to the work of Isabel Menzies Lyth, and how professionals defend themselves from intolerable affects. I suggest that the eradication of difference between forensic professional and patient generates enormous fear and rage in other professionals and it is these affects that 'blind' other professionals to what is going on with one of their colleagues.

There is also the question of how the professional involved (literally) loses 'sight' of the boundary between themselves and the patient and what they lose sight of. In my (limited) involvement in cases of sexual boundary violations by staff, I have been struck by how blind the staff members have been to the danger they were in; not just professionally but personally. It is as if they have not let themselves 'see' the 'cruel and unusual' part of the patient, or what might better called 'dark matter' because it is presumed to fill the space that is each person's moral universe. In one case I am aware of, a nurse shut herself in an enclosed space with a patient who had previously made a severe and near-fatal assault on a woman *with whom he had an acquaintance*. When the original victim went to meet him, her idea of what might happen between them bore no relationship to what he had planned for her. In the same way, the staff member had no idea of what was in this patient's mind when they hid together.

This event did not end in tragedy but it could have. I can only speculate that the nurse was 'blinded' by some other affect: anger and excitement at rule-breaking? Unconscious suicidality? An unconscious but desperate need for their own care? In this case (as in so many) there is no testimony from the professional in question except for that constructed for the disciplinary and legal action afterwards, which understandably denies guilt or attempts to shift responsibility elsewhere. In this particular case, I was also interested to note that the other staff on duty had a 'feeling' or an 'idea' where their colleague was but could not bear to look.

CONCLUSION

The earliest research on sexual misconduct by psychiatrists and psychotherapists was published in 1977, and it is said (and sad if true) that these first researchers were threatened with professional disciplinary procedures for researching this subject. The first British book on this subject was not published until 1994 (Holmes and Lindley 1994). There is still no formal study of sexual boundary violations by forensic professionals nor of boundary violations in forensic settings more generally, despite four high-profile public inquiries into abuses of care in high secure facilities.

No amount of codes of conduct or mandatory training will prevent a disturbed and unhappy person embarking on a dangerous course of action, whether they are currently patients or professionals. In forensic work, we need to continue to help each other to ask, 'What am I not thinking about?' This question, with its paradoxical quality, does not expect an answer, only the readiness to admit that we do not know, and cannot be certain. In forensic settings, we need to teach ourselves to be uncertain about safety and risk but certain about dignity and respect for all parties. My position would be that we need to assume that the dark matter is always there and that the work for forensic psychiatric services is to help the patient deal with it better. This entails the assumption that we ourselves will be touched by the dark matter of the patient's mind and we need to continually explore it in reflective and supervisory spaces.

REFERENCES

Adshead, G. (1998) 'Psychiatric staff as attachment figures: understanding management problems in psychiatric service in the light of attachment theory.' *British Journal of Psychiatry 172*, 64–69.

Aiyegbusi, A. and Clarke-Moore, J. (2009) *Therapeutic relationships with offenders: An Introduction to the Psychodynamics of Forensic Mental Health Nursing.* London: Jessica Kingsley Publishers.

Bernal, E. (1992) 'The Nurse as Patient Advocate.' *Hastings Center Report 22*, 4, 18–23.

Bowlby, J. (1970) 'Disruption of affectional bonds and its effect on behaviour.' *Journal of Contemporary Psychotherapy 2*, 2, 75–86.

Bowlby, J. (1977) 'The making and breaking of affectional bonds; aetiology and psychopathology in light of attachment theory.' *British Journal of Psychiatry 130*, 201–210.

Coid, J. (1992) 'DSM-II diagnoses in criminal psychopaths: a way forward.' *Criminal Behaviour and Mental Health 2*, 78–94.

Cox, M. (1988) *Structuring the therapeutic process: Compromise with chaos.* London: Jessica Kingsley Publishers.

Daffern, M., Jones, L. and Shine, J. (2010) *Offence paralleling behaviour: a case formulation approach to offender assessment and intervention.* Chichester: John Wiley.

Dozier M., Lomax, L., Tyrrell, C. and Lee, S. (2001) 'The challenge of treatment for clients with dismissing states of mind.' *Attachment and Human Development 3*, 1, 62–76.

Eastman, N. (1999) 'Public health psychiatry or crime prevention?' *British Medical Journal 318*, 549.

Frese, F.J. III, Stanley, J., Kress, K. and Vogel-Scibilia, S. (2001) 'Interpreting evidence based practices and the recovery model.' *Psychiatric Services 52*, 1462–1468.

Gabbard, G. (ed.) (1989) *Sexual exploitation in professional relationships.* Washington, DC: American Psychiatric Press.

Henderson, S. (1974) 'Care eliciting behaviour in man.' *Journal of Nervous and Mental Disease 159*, 172–181.

Holmes, J. and Lindley, R. (1994) 'Ethics and Psychotherapy.' In R. Gillon (ed.) *Principles of Health Care Ethics.* Chichester: John Wiley.

Kessler, R., McLaughlin, K., Grief Green, J., Gruber, M.J., *et al.* (2010) 'Childhood adversities and adult psychopathology in the WHO World Mental Health Survey.' *British Journal of Psychiatry 197*, 378–385.

Kleinman, A. (2009) 'Caregiving: the odyssey of becoming more human.' *The Lancet 373*, 292–293.

Kluft, R.P. (1990) 'Sequela of incest: therapist–patient sexual exploitation with a description of the sitting duck syndrome.' In R.P. Kluft (ed.) *Incest related syndrome of adult psychopathology.* Arlington VA: American Psychiatric Press.

Latane, B. and Darley J.M. (1970) *The unresponsive bystander: Why doesn't he help?* New York: Appleton-Century-Crofts.

Lowdell, A. and Adshead, G. (2009) 'The best defence: institutional defences against anxiety in forensic services.' In A. Aiyegbusi and J. Clarke-Moore (eds) *Therapeutic Relationships with Offenders: An Introduction to the Psychodynamics of Forensic Mental Health Nursing.* London: Jessica Kingsley Publishers.

Main, T. (1957) 'The Ailment.' *British Journal of Medical Psychology 30*, 129–145.

Menzies Lyth, I. (1988) *Containing Anxiety in Institutions: Selected essays. Volume 1.* London: Free Association Books.

Okai, D., Owen, G., McGuire, H. and Singh, S. (2007) 'Mental capacity in psychiatric patients: a systematic review.' *British Journal of Psychiatry 191*, 291–297.

Robinson, D. and Kettles, A. (1999) *Forensic nursing and multidisciplinary care of the mentally disordered offender.* London: Jessica Kingsley Publishers.

Sapolsky, R. (2004) 'Social status in humans and other animals.' *Annual Review of Anthropology 33*, 393–418.

Sarkar, S. (2004) 'Boundary violation and sexual exploitation in psychiatry: A review.' *Advances in Psychiatric Treatment 10*, 312–320.

Schore, A.N. (1994) *Affect Regulation and the Origin of the Self. The Neurobiology of Emotional Development.* Hillsdale, NJ: Lawrence Erlbaum.

Steiner, J. (1985) 'Turning a blind eye: the cover up for Oedipus.' *International Review of Psychoanalysis 12*, 161–172.

Szasz, T. (1989) *Law, liberty and psychiatry: an inquiry into the social uses of mental health practice.* New York: University of Syracuse Press.

Thomas-Peter, B. and Garrett, T. (2000) 'Preventing sexual contact between professional and patients in forensic environments.' *Journal of Forensic Psychiatry 11*, 135–150.

van IJzendoorn, M.H. and Bakermans Kranenburg, M. (2008) 'The distribution of adult attachment representations in clinical groups: a meta analytic search for patterns of attachment in 105 AAI studies.' In H. Steele and M. Steele (eds) *Clinical Applications of the Adult Attachment Interview.* New York: Guilford.

Veatch, R. (1972) 'Models for Ethical Medicine in a Revolutionary Age.' *Hastings Center Report* 2, 3, 5–7.

Veatch, R. (2000) *Cross cultural perspectives in medical ethics*. London: Jones and Bartlett.

Chapter 2

THE PATIENT'S EXPERIENCE OF PROFESSIONAL ABUSE IN THE PSYCHOLOGICAL THERAPIES

Dawn Devereux

Overview

While psychological therapy, like any effective treatment, can bring great benefits to patients, there is also strong evidence that it can cause considerable harm (Jarrett 2008). The aim of this chapter is to bring the patient's experience of iatrogenic harm to life, so that mental health professionals may appreciate that very real and lasting damage can result from the violation of professional boundaries. There are a number of seminal works on the subject from the USA (Gabbard and Lester 1995; Pope and Vasquez 2001; Schoener *et al.* 1989) but very little literature from the UK. This chapter will therefore offer a predominantly UK perspective and will concentrate on those aspects of professional abuse that may be commonly misunderstood by professionals.

INTRODUCTION

In order to present the patient's perspective, experiential accounts will be referred to, taken from the growing literature on abusive professional relationships. These accounts are all available in the public domain and so enable authentic, verbatim experience to be conveyed without the concerns about confidentiality that are required when clinical material is used. This will be supplemented, throughout the chapter, by the more general experience of clients who have sought help from the Clinic for Boundaries Studies (CfBS), the only specialist psychotherapy and support service for the survivors of professional abuse in the UK. Since the chapter makes extensive use of the client literature, I will begin by describing this genre.

THE CLIENT LITERATURE

First-person accounts of negative effects from psychological therapy started to appear in the middle years of the last century when several psychoanalysts wrote about their own damaging experience of psychoanalysis (Little 1951; Rycroft 1995). Published lay accounts only began at the end of the 1970s with Freeman and Roy's (1976) book *Betrayal*, followed a few years later by Ellen Plasil's (1985) *Therapist* and Carolyn Bates and Annette Brodsky's (1989) *Sex in the Therapy Hour*. Although early lay accounts all came from the USA, there is now also an extensive client-authored literature emerging from the UK.

These accounts have not generally been welcomed by the professions and have attracted predominantly negative reviews in professional journals. The degree of hostility is best exemplified by the lampooning nature of many of the reviews. For example, Lena Davis' (1996) review of Rosie Alexander's book *Folie a Deux* (Alexander and Spinelli 1999) was given the mocking title 'Rosie in Horrorland', while client accounts in *Shouldn't I be Feeling Better by Now?* (Bates 2006) were dismissed by the psychotherapist Louise Guy (2006, p.42) in *Therapy Today* as 'an anti-therapy tirade'. She found none of the client accounts to be of any value and seemed genuinely bemused that anyone would think them worth reading.

PREVALENCE OF ABUSE

As mentioned in the overview, there is a general perception that abuse by psychological therapists is rare, so it seems important to begin by addressing the question of prevalence. This is notoriously difficult to estimate because both professionals and patients are generally unwilling to disclose abuse. Whilst most professionals do not admit (even anonymously) to perpetrating abuse, there is evidence that many fail to recognise that aspects of their own behaviour are abusive (Epstein, Simon and Kay 1995). As a result, figures on professional abuse tend to greatly underestimate the problem. Both the client literature and consultations undertaken at the CfBS show that very few people who have experienced professional abuse make a formal complaint. This is not because clients do not feel harmed; in the majority of cases they simply feel too depleted by the exploitation to complain. In addition, complaints processes (especially under self-regulation) can be notoriously difficult to negotiate and many organisations are hostile to complainants, as illustrated by the following client's experience:

> I was so incapacitated by the abuse and the complaints process was so intimidating that I never got past the first hurdle which was phoning the institution he belonged to. I said I wanted him to be accountable and the woman I spoke to said 'you sound very angry and revengeful' – that was the end of that. (Pearson 2002, p.2)

It is important to note, with regard to prevalence, that abusive professionals are disproportionately found to be experienced practitioners who are highly regarded by colleagues (Gabbard and Lester 1995); they may also have held positions on ethics committees (Levine 2010). It is necessary to be explicit about this, as clients who contact the CfBS often report that the high standing of the professional has made them doubt their own experience and has also prevented them from making their experience known.

Conservative estimates concerning the prevalence of sexual abuse within professional relationships puts the figure at around five per cent, with a consensus amongst leading commentators that the true figure will be far in excess (Gabbard and Lester 1995; Pope and Vasquez 2001; Schoener *et al.* 1989). This figure rises considerably when considering non-sexual boundary violations. Epstein *et al.* (1995) found that when asking therapists to consider an index of boundary violations, 43 per cent of respondents indicated that there was at least one item that alerted them to an exploitative aspect of their own practice. Empirical studies on patients' experiences of psychotherapy show that between 12 per cent and 33 per cent of clients have negative outcomes (Crown 1983; Henry, Sims and Spray 1971; Shapiro 1976). These figures, combined with under-reporting, make it evident that iatrogenic harm is a serious problem.

CLIENT PROFILES AND BEHAVIOURS

Various myths have emerged in relation to the type of people who are likely to experience professional abuse and so it seems important to address this question directly. Clients from all walks of life experience boundary violations and social, intellectual or professional status is no bar to experiencing abusive actions or their effects. The literature evidences (among others) full-time mothers, teachers, authors, journalists, economists, psychiatrists, psychotherapists, lawyers, academics and nurses as victims of professional abuse.

In terms of the psychological and personality profile of patients who are harmed, it is clear that people who have had difficult attachment histories are more at risk. It is important to stress, however, that they are not more likely to experience professional exploitation per se; they are simply more likely to be profoundly affected by it. This is because the abusive relationship may be experienced as a repetition of developmental trauma. An additional reason, is that such patients often develop an idealising transference[1] because they long for a secure attachment figure. As a result they may (unconsciously) project all of the longed-for parental characteristics onto the therapist, who is then experienced as being uniquely capable of meeting their needs (Devereux 2010). While most therapists will interpret this phenomenon, in order to empower the patient, therapists operating from a more narcissistic position often encourage the patient's idealisation and dependency in the interests of their own ego.

A patient, Dr K, caught up in this kind of idealisation, explains the allure of the relationship particularly succinctly:

> …a thirst never quenched was now being slaked. And perhaps most important, I felt it was being slaked by him. Not by the process. Not by something in me… (Gabbard and Lester 1995, p.132)

If the professional is idealised it may be especially difficult for the patient to acknowledge abusive behaviour, because this will threaten the idealisation. Patient accounts show that the two most common strategies for dealing with this are self-blame and attempts to repair the professional. As one client wrote: 'Although he began to undermine and pathologise me, I couldn't face up to what was happening because I was so dependent on him, if I accepted the fault was with me I didn't have to face losing him' (Pearson 2002, p.3). It is important for professionals to understand this dynamic because patients are often unjustly criticised for failing to leave an abusive professional relationship.

SEXUAL BOUNDARY VIOLATIONS: THE EFFECTS AND MISUNDERSTANDINGS

In terms of the consequences of sexual contact, there is a consensus in the literature that the effects of professional sexual abuse are likely to be profound.

---

1   Transference is a psychoanalytic concept that refers to the fact that we all transfer feelings and longings about significant people from the past onto people in the present. An idealising transference is most likely to occur when someone has longed for a secure parent and so projects that longing onto the professional and experiences that person in a distorted way.

For example, in Luepker's (1999) study of clients who had been sexually involved with professionals, 95 per cent met the criteria for post-traumatic stress disorder. In a similar study Somer and Nachmanil (2005) found that all respondents described high levels of dependence, confusion and dissociation. At the CfBS we find that clients experience a range of different, often very ambivalent, emotions ranging from rage and suicidal ideation to guilt and concern for the perpetrator. In addition they may suffer from an overwhelming sense of anxiety, loss of confidence, plummeting self-esteem and confusion. This is sometimes also accompanied by a profound feeling of shame.

Shame often leads to isolation, not least because patients feel that their experience is not understood. Friends, relatives and even professionals frequently confuse the non-coercive nature of most sexual abuse by professionals with consent and so may feel that the patient is partly, or even equally, responsible. Transference issues, the power relationship, the knowledge differential, 'duty of care' and the need to trust professionals make the consent of a patient to sexual relations no more legitimate than the consent of a child. Patients who consult the CfBS frequently report that mental health professionals, to whom they are referred for further treatment, describe their abuse as an 'affair' and tell them it is no different from the end of any romantic relationship. This is extremely unhelpful and confusing for the patient.

Unlike childhood sexual abuse, which is a frequently discussed topic of conversation in the media, there is little public discourse on the subject of professional sexual abuse and abused patients often feel profoundly alone and are likely to struggle to find a vocabulary to describe their experience (Devereux 2011). The restorative effect of discovering such a discourse is evidenced by the fact that CfBS clients often describe this as a crucial part of their recovery.

Collateral damage to family members is also an under-recognised effect of professional abuse. A therapist writing anonymously about her training therapy stated:

> …seduced by the raptures of merger, I was numb to the pain I was causing my husband, and to my own pain at the physical separation from him and the emotional distance from my children… (Anonymous 2005, p.671)

Another client wrote:

> I cannot over-emphasize the devastating effect all this had on my husband and children. I think they could not recognise the person they had known – a family orientated wife and mother. It was as if an alien had invaded my being and I was speaking and behaving in ways that were just not me. (Matheson 2008, p.57)

NON-SEXUAL EXPLOITATION: AN UNDER-RECOGNISED CAUSE OF PROFOUND HARM

Experts in the field warn against taking a hierarchical approach that assumes that certain violations are inherently more damaging than others (Gabbard and Lester 1995). Emotional abuse by a professional may seem less shocking and graphic than sexual abuse but it can be just as insidiously damaging and undermining. The majority of calls to the CfBS are about non-sexual boundary violations, and we do not find any discernible difference between sexual and non-sexual exploitation in terms of effects on the client.

The degree to which lax boundaries can cause profound and intractable anxiety is not generally appreciated. Joan Riviere's experience with the psychoanalyst Ernest Jones illustrates this particularly well. Jones, apparently, would: give no regular appointment time; confide his marital problems; let Riviere stay in his summer cottage; and ask for her help with academic translations (Schwartz 1999). Though such actions may not make it into codes of ethics, Riviere suffered greatly. Her colleagues noticed how her confidence plummeted and she eventually became so anxious and withdrawn that she was unable to speak at meetings of the London Psychoanalytic Society (Schwartz 1999). Lax appointment times and personal disclosures are commonly reported to the CfBS and our clients corroborate the experience of Riviere in terms of a resulting loss of confidence and profound anxiety.

In my own previous analysis of actions that produce negative effects in psychotherapy (Devereux 2011), four distinct categories emerged, as shown in Table 2.1. One of the most important findings from this research was that the knowledge differential was a persistent factor in almost all exploitation. Although this could be active exploitation through actions such as pathologising, false logic and unwarranted certainty, it was also found to work passively by imbuing all of the professional's actions with a legitimacy that it is difficult for patients to challenge. As a result, any discursive act, from inviting a sexual relationship to disclosing personal information, can become imbued with an unwarranted legitimacy. This makes the knowledge differential a seminal factor in almost all instances of professional abuse.

Table 2.1 Actions that lead to negative effects in psychological therapy	
Category	Sub-category
KNOWINGLY misusing professional knowledge	Pathologising
	Certainty
	Disempowering language
	False logic
	Determining the process of therapy
	Refusing negative feedback
	Imposing values
	Withholding information
EXPLOITING the therapeutic process	Mishandling the idealising transference
	Encouraging dependency
	Inappropriately breaking down defences
	Recapitulating developmental trauma
	Interfering with real life
	Termination difficulties
PERVERTING the therapeutic space	Sexual contact
	Sexualised discourse
	Physical violence
	Aggressive verbal attacks
	Cruel/mocking humour
	Sadism
DEPRIVING the client of the therapeutic space	Irrelevant disclosure
	Personal preoccupations
	Reacting
	Inadequate attention
	Arriving late
	Taking phone calls
	Falling asleep
	Failing to engage with client's agenda

In its active form, the pathologising of clients was shown to be particularly prevalent and, again, is often reported by clients who contact the CfBS. It may take the form of a 'diagnosis' – psychotic, borderline and personality disordered being the most common – or as undermining comments such as telling clients they are shallow, not worthwhile, of no interest, boring, inherently bad, sadistic, stupid, underdeveloped, immoral, an abuser or a loser. The journalist Virginia Ironside describes various therapists telling her that she was:

> …aggressive, hostile, in denial, manipulative, unhelpable. I was weird, somehow inhuman, different. (Ironside 2006, p.1)

The pathologising of patients is a particularly insidious form of abuse because it profoundly disempowers and depletes patients, leaving them more susceptible to further abuse. Patients find pathologising discourse very difficult to refute because it is inextricably tied to the professional's expert knowledge.

Clients who consult the CfBS suggest that this kind of pathologising often intensifies in the final session, especially when clients are leaving the therapy without the agreement of the professional. In cases of NHS treatment it may occur where a patient has declined the suggestion that they continue to see the professional privately. Patients commonly report that abusive verbal treatment in the final session (often experienced as a revenge attack) is particularly likely to be internalised and can become a major impediment to recovery.

Before concluding, it seems important to draw attention to one of the most under-recognised effects of professional abuse (whether sexual or non-sexual): its intractable and persistent nature. This is evidenced by the fact that a high number of calls to the CfBS are from people who were abused by a professional over a decade ago, and sometimes much longer. Many survivors have never told anyone about their experience and most assumed that the effects would eventually dissipate. This is frequently not the case, especially when patients have never spoken about the abuse, as exemplified by the following client, disclosing the abuse for the first time sixteen years after her abusive treatment ended:

> When it eventually ended I experienced a great feeling of relief and though still extremely upset I assumed the impact would fade. It never did – it intensified and would descend on me in confusing and unpredictable ways: profound, devastating sadness, intense rage, unbearable feelings of badness but always, always, unrelenting isolation, utter confusion and no means of expressing my experience or feelings in a way that could be understood by anyone. (Rooks 2002, p.3)

CONCLUSION

This chapter has employed client accounts and the experience of the CfBS to provide a predominantly UK perspective on the client's experience of professional abuse. Most mental health professionals will be aware of exploitative practices at some time in their careers, either directly from patients or through observation or hearsay. This chapter has emphasised the importance of treating such information in the most serious possible way. By presenting the patient's perspective and concentrating on aspects of professional abuse that are commonly misunderstood, my aim has been to encourage practitioners to respond to patients in an empathic and proactive manner whenever they become aware of exploitative practice.

REFERENCES

Alexander, R. and Spinelli, E. (1995) *Folie a Deux: An Experience of One-to-One Therapy.* London: Free Association Books.

Anonymous (2005) 'The unfolding and healing of analytic boundary violations: personal, clinical and cultural considerations.' *Journal of Analytical Psychology 50,* 661–691.

Bates, C. and Brodsky, A. (1989) *Sex in the Therapy Hour: A Case of Professional Incest.* New York: Guildford Press.

Bates, Y. (ed.) (2006) *Shouldn't I be Feeling Better by Now? Client Views of Therapy.* London: Palgrave Macmillan.

Crown, S. (1983) 'Contraindications and dangers of psychotherapy.' *British Journal of Psychiatry 143,* 436–441.

Davis, L. (1996) 'Rosie in Horrorland: Review of Alexander's *Folie a Deux.*' *Counselling News 30.*

Devereux, D. (2010) 'The Patient's Perspective.' In F. Subotsky, M. Crowe and S. Bewley (eds) *Abuse of the Doctor Patient Relationship: Current issues.* London: Royal College of Psychiatrists.

Devereux, D. (2011) 'A grounded theory exploration of actions that give rise to negative effects in psychological therapies: the client's perspective.' In preparation.

Epstein, R., Simon, R. and Kay, G. (1995) 'Bulletin of the Menninger Clinic LVI, 1992, Assessing Boundary Violations in Psychotherapy: Survey Results with the Exploitation Index.' *Psychoanal Quarterly 64,* 635–636.

Freeman, L. and Roy, J. (1976) *Betrayal: The true story of the first woman to successfully sue her psychiatrist for using sex in the guise of therapy.* New York: Stein and Day.

Gabbard, G. and Lester, E. (1995) *Boundaries and Boundary Violations in Psychoanalysis.* New York: Basic Books.

Guy, L. (2006) Book review: 'Shouldn't I be feeling better by now?' *Therapy Today 17,* 8, p.51.

Henry, W., Sims, J. and Spray, S. (1971) *The Fifth Profession.* San Francisco: Jossey-Bass.

Ironside, V. (2006) 'Anti-therapy.' In Y. Bates (ed.) *Shouldn't I be Feeling Better by Now?* London: Palgrave Macmillan.

Jarrett, C. (2008) 'When therapy causes harm.' *The Psychologist 21,* 1, 10–12.

Levine, H. (2010) 'Sexual Boundary Violations: A Psychoanalytic Perspective.' *British Journal of Psychotherapy 26*, 1, 50–63.

Little, M. (1951) 'Counter-Transference and the Patient's Response to It.' *International Journal of Psychoanalysis 21*.

Luepker, E. (1999) 'Effects of practitioners' sexual misconduct: A follow up study.' *Journal of the American Academy of Psychiatry and the Law 27*, 1, 51–63.

Matheson, M. (2008) 'Broken Boundaries.' In S. Richardson and M. Cunningham (eds) *Broken Boundaries*. London: Witness.

Pearson, S. (2002) 'Paying to be Tortured.' *Survivors' Forum 1*, 1, 2–8.

Plasil, E. (1985) *Therapist*. New York, NY: St. Martin's/Marek.

Pope, K. and Vasquez, M. (2001) *Ethics in Psychotherapy and Counselling: A Practical Guide* (2nd edn). San Francisco: Jossey-Bass.

Rooks, R. (Spring 2002) 'Keep me Safe.' *Survivors' Forum 1*, 2, 2–7.

Rycroft, C. (1995) 'Reminiscences of a survivor: psychoanalysis 1937–1993.' *British Journal of Psychotherapy 11*, 4, 514–521.

Schoener, G., Milgrom, J., Gonsiorek, J., Luepker, E. and Conroe, R. (1989) *Psychotherapists' Sexual Involvement with Clients: Intervention and Prevention*. Chicago: Walk-in Counselling Center.

Schwartz, J. (1999) *Cassandra's Daughter*. London: Penguin Books.

Shapiro, D. (1976) 'The analyst's analysis.' *Journal of the American Psychoanalytic Association 24*, 5–42.

Somer, E. and Nachmanil, I. (2005) 'Constructions of therapist-client sex: A comparative analysis of retrospective victim reports.' *Sexual Abuse: Journal of Research and Treatment 17*, 1, 47–62.

Chapter 3

BOUNDARY VIOLATIONS: ARE TRANSGRESSING PROFESSIONALS BEYOND HELP?

Jonathan Coe and Glen Gabbard

Overview

The UK lags behind the USA in terms of professional and regulatory understanding of the risk and rehabilitation potentials of professionals who have been found to have violated professional boundaries with their patients (Coe 2010; Snowden 2010). For some decades American specialists (Gabbard 1989; Gabbard and Myers 2008; Schoener 1989) have taken the view that it is possible for some practitioners to successfully undergo rehabilitation programs and arrive at a position where clinical and regulatory authorities make an assessment that their risk to patients is minimal. These practitioners may then be subject to long-term monitoring and have strict conditions placed on their practice. The aim of this chapter is to highlight key issues from the experience of Professor Glen Gabbard at The Gabbard Center, an international center of expertise based in Houston, Texas. This will be achieved through an interview with Professor Gabbard which is conducted by Jonathan Coe, Managing Director for the Clinic for Boundary Studies in the United Kingdom.

INTRODUCTION

In the USA there are a range of services providing specialist evaluation, rehabilitation or educational services for professionals who have transgressed professional boundaries. These services typically deal with a range of different professions, including health workers, clergy and psychological practitioners. Whilst some services use a model of treatment stemming from work with sex offenders, many are informed by an understanding of psychodynamic processes. One such is led by Professor Glen Gabbard, Clinical Professor of Psychiatry at Baylor College of Medicine in Houston, Texas, and a founder of The Gabbard Center. He is also the author of *Boundaries and Boundary Violations in Psychoanalysis and Physician as Patient: A Clinical Handbook for Mental Health Professionals*. The Gabbard Center provides three-day multi-disciplinary evaluations of professionals accused of boundary violations, most often involving sexualization of the relationship, but also including financial and other transgressions. The Center assesses about equal numbers of priests, physicians and talking therapists. The majority of those assessed have either a psychiatric condition on Axis 1 of the DSM, a personality disorder, or both. Sometimes they have personality traits that do not reach the threshold for a disorder but account for some of their behaviors. The clinic also sees people who are psychologically healthy but under tremendous stress.

JC *Do you have a structured approach in terms of assessing the individual's potential for risk and rehabilitation?*

GG Psychological testing is very structured, there's a whole series of standard instruments, but in my interviews I rely more on open-ended questions and my sense of where the midline is in terms of responses, and what are the outliers. The question would be: "Is this person amenable to rehabilitation?" Some are and some aren't. One of the things I look for in my evaluations is this: "Do they get it: do they get the problem?" A lot of them say things like, "The other guys working in the hospital are so much worse than I am." The other thing is to see if there is any real genuine remorse. In my writing one of the points I make is that there's a difference between narcissistic mortification on the one hand, and genuine remorse on the other. I'll ask an open-ended question: "Do you feel bad about what's happened?" Some of the professionals respond by saying, "Do I feel bad? Are you kidding? My life is destroyed, my family is disgraced, my career is destroyed. If I could rewind the tape I would never do this again." And in all of this they haven't mentioned the victim one time. When I ask about harm to the victim, the same professional may say, "I suppose that's possible, I've read about it. But this woman was really very interested in a sexual relationship – I don't think she was harmed by it, this was what she wanted." This is another example of not getting it, or being so narcissistic and self-absorbed they can only see their own situation. They are manifesting a problem with mentalizing – they can't mentalize the response of the victim, how that person would feel. That's another bad sign, because they're likely to be at high risk for recurrence. So we try to assess – do they get it, are they genuinely remorseful, are they at high risk for recurrence? For some people we say we don't think it's a good idea even to go into a rehabilitation program, and we suggest going into a different profession. It's very difficult to do with the person sitting there, but I've done it a number of times. Often they're expecting it.

JC *Are you mandated to report where the person admits additional offences?*

GG It goes in the report and generally the referrer will report it. There's a certain percentage of people who will break down – I look them in the eye and say, "Are you really telling me the whole truth? Are you really being completely honest with me?" And there's a percentage who get tearful and say, "Well, there's another victim."

JC *I'm wondering if the places that run treatment programs are treating, as a boundary violation is not a medical condition?*

GG I think they are often treating the defense of denial. But I'm talking about three to five years of rehabilitation – a program that goes on and is monitored for years. Usually there's no need for inpatient or residential. The programs we set up are independent, to some degree, of disciplinary systems. Boards may get in touch and say, "We've suspended this person for 18 months, but we'd like you to see him and determine if it would be worthwhile to set up a treatment and rehabilitation programme." So here's a typical program: individual psychotherapy every week with someone who understands professional boundaries; an educational seminar and restriction on practice – for example if the clinician has been in solo practice, he or she needs to work in an institution or a group under supervision. We also might recommend that they go over prospective patients with a mentor or supervisor, who helps them screen out certain patients, such as those with childhood trauma histories.

Sometimes marital therapy is helpful, and sometimes medication is needed if they're very depressed. Those would be the major components. Then the total program needs to be monitored for three to five years. Before they can practice outside the monitoring program, they need to be re-evaluated to see if they grasp what they have done, that is, do they "get it." Many of them do. I think when they're carefully selected, many of these people can be rehabilitated quite well, especially those who've had a lovesick situation where the infatuation wears off during the three to five years and they think, "I was acting irrationally, what was I thinking of; I love my spouse or partner, why did I do this?" So the good news is that many improve substantially. Maybe half we see have good potential for rehabilitation. That's an estimate but roughly what I would think. Someone who would never be recommended for a treatment or rehab program is the person who says "I didn't do it." To construct a program for such a person has an inherent absurdity in it: rehabilitation for what? I also say: "This isn't a courtroom, I'm not a private detective. I can't determine whether you did or didn't do it. I'm just a psychiatrist trying to evaluate whether you have any emotional problems." So I get out of trying to be judge and jury, or tricking them into saying anything. Most are admitting something by the time they get to me.

JC *You have been very clear that often the issue is not black and white and that an understanding of the complexities of each case is vital. I am interested in whether, ethically, there are some practitioners who simply shouldn't be rehabilitated?*

GG Absolutely. That's why I estimated that only 50 per cent are likely to do well in rehabilitation. There are severe narcissistic personality disorders and sociopathic therapists who are essentially predators. They have no remorse for their transgressions. This is why a careful evaluation with substantial collateral information is needed to assess who can be rehabilitated and who cannot be rehabilitated.

JC *What about long-term monitoring?*

GG I learned the hard way that there has to be someone responsible for doing this. If it's up to the practitioner himself, nothing will happen. Church authorities, licensing boards, and physician health organizations may require that the professional have regular drug or alcohol screenings. An appointed rehabilitation coordinator, whether in a licensing board, hospital, or church diocese, will get a regular one-line letter from the treating therapist which confirms that the person is attending treatment and thereby completing that part of the plan. We think that the content of the therapy must be confidential or the therapy can be a "sham therapy" where the patient is concealing what he or she is doing. Only attendance is revealed to the monitor. In some cases a monitor from a licensing board may pay a visit to the doctor's office to see about the chaperoning practices or examine medical records.

VICTIMS

JC *Sometimes the issue of Sexual Boundary Violation is taken as a kind of technical breach, an offence to good manners – could you give a perspective on the ethical basis for its proscription and something of what is established about harm to clients?*

GG The essence of a fiduciary relationship where one pays another for a service is beneficence and non-maleficence. The relationship exists to help the patient. Non-maleficence refers to the time-honored principle of "First, do no harm." So sexual exploitation is unethical in many ways. First, it is a rip-off. One comes for therapy and instead receives sex. The problems that brought the person to therapy go unaddressed. Moreover, there is a power differential built into the therapeutic relationship by virtue of one person paying another who has a specific expertise. It is difficult to say "no" to a more powerful person who has special expertise that you need. Hence it is an abuse of power and a situation where one cannot give informed consent. There is ample evidence from clinical studies that patients feel harmed, betrayed, and may be refractory to subsequent treatment since they cannot trust future therapists. Some may not complain initially if they are in love with the therapist or marry the therapist, but that love is temporally unstable in most instances, and there is rage when the relationship goes sour. This is what Gutheil and I call cessation trauma (Gabbard and Gutheil 1992).

JC *What about the rules governing former clients?*

GG Different states and different professional organizations have different policies on post-termination boundaries. However, I think that what is unethical during treatment is generally going to be unethical after treatment. In one case a woman said to her therapist, "Are you attracted to me?" and "I know you're going to a meeting, and I would like to meet you there, are you attracted to me?" The therapist responded, "That would be highly unethical, for now this relationship has to be purely therapy." She told me she hung on to those words "for now" and she said that therapy stopped from that moment on because all she could think about was "for now." That means "at some future point he may want me." For the rest of her therapy she didn't talk about her problems – she tried to be an attractive enticing woman to increase her chances of a romantic relationship. So she wasn't doing therapy anymore – she was trying to seduce him.

When there is an arbitrary time limit, for example two years post-termination, on sexual contact, the therapy stops working. The patient thinks, "I won't mention any sexual problems because he may not want to date me in two years, I'll keep quiet about all this." I always make the point to my students that the reason the therapy works is that you are once and forever only a therapist for the patient. Once the patient understands that you will never be anything but a therapist, then he or she can really open up because there are no consequences in any other relationship. Once you depart from that you're in trouble. That's the reason why it makes sense to me to have an ethics code that says "once a patient always a patient" so the patient then thinks "there's no hope here for anything else so I might as well be open and tell everything about myself."

JC *Could you expand on the ways in which non-sexual boundaries are breached, and the consequences of this for the patient?*

GG There are many, many ways that non-sexual boundaries are breached. I will cite just a few: gossiping about a patient, making a business deal with a patient, soliciting a donation from a patient, asking a patient to babysit one's kids or work in the office, or telling the patient you are in love with him/her. The patient is harmed because for therapy to work, it has to be clear that the patient is there only for treatment and for no other purpose. Non-sexual boundary violations place the therapist's needs before the patient's. Moreover, patients who are told "I love you" or are treated as friends have false hope raised that they will be something other than a patient for the therapist.

JC *Do you see people who've been abused by practitioners?*

GG Yes, as therapy patients. Sometimes a victim will come to me and want to make a complaint. Historically the victims have been neglected, that is, they have not been taken seriously. One of the things I also have done before is mediation, sitting down with both the professional and the victim. Getting the therapist to apologize can be tremendously important for the victim. I've also negotiated within mediation the return of the fees by the therapist to the patient. Some of the practitioners feel they haven't done anything wrong, so they don't want to apologize or explain. They blame the victim. I've had a mediation situation where the practitioner expressed his anger at the patient for ruining his career. It took several sessions for him to see that it wasn't just him who had been harmed. It turned out pretty well. He had to listen to the damage he'd done. Mediation is not right for everyone but it's good to have options available.

RISK FACTORS AND TYPES OF TRANSGRESSOR

JC *What is known about practitioners who violate boundaries?*

GG A whole spectrum of different people do this for different reasons. I'm convinced that people hate complexity – they like to say: "All of these guys are bad, they're evil, they're predators, let's throw them out, throw the bad apple out of the barrel, then everything will be fine." But it doesn't work that way. My students sometimes say: "Why are you teaching us this, Professor Gabbard? This is nothing I'm ever going to do, so why will I ever need to know about this?" So yes, everybody's vulnerable and people who think they'll never get in trouble are the people who may get in trouble because they're not thinking about it. Every one of us is a master of self-deception. If you're working alone in a private office somewhere, without consultation, you can convince yourself "I'm an exception. This isn't in any way exploitative, it's true love, there's nothing wrong with this." So I teach that if you're going to be a therapist for the rest of your life, you need a supervisor or consultant. You internalize a consultant and carry that person into the room with you, so you're having a dialogue in your mind. That's the best prevention.

Isolation, the solo practitioner working alone, is a high-risk situation, as there is a boundary problem built into that. You tend to drift away from what is accepted practice if you're totally by yourself. Practitioners more advanced in their careers who think they don't need to consult or to continue to learn and grow may be at high risk as well, especially if they are in solo practice. Many practitioners I've seen are well-respected teachers and supervisors. I have so many examples of the narcissistic guy who's well known in the field who says: "Well, you know, the rules don't really apply to me anymore, because I know what I'm doing. If one of my supervisees did this I'd be worried about it, but *I* know what I'm doing, so I can get away with it." Or "I'm unorthodox, people wouldn't understand. I couldn't talk to a supervisor because they wouldn't understand my approach – I've done it with lots of people and it's different but it works." Narcissism is a huge problem in the mental health field.

JC *With psychological therapists, have you determined any differences between modalities in terms of clinical profile or in how transgressions play out?*

GG No, therapists of all persuasions are vulnerable. It has much more to do with the particular characteristics of the patient and therapist than any particular theory, technique or modality.

JC *Are the majority of people that you see one-time offenders?*

GG Yes, but we see multiple offenders too. I'd say maybe 60 per cent are one-time offenders.

JC *How about those who are not the long-term predators of dozens of victims but may have two, four, six victims?*

GG These practitioners may be narcissistically organized. Many are womanizers, but haven't been doing it with patients. The guy who fancies himself a Don Juan, lots of girlfriends, several wives. But one patient, and that's why he gets sent to me. Those who have only one victim are often superego-ridden, obsessive compulsive. They have always done everything the right way, and they have a kind of mid-life crisis. They may think, "My God I've done everything by the book my whole life – I deserve one little transgression with one patient. For once I'm going to throw off the shackles of oppressive orthodoxy, I've earned it."

EPIDEMIOLOGY AND DENIAL

JC *The research into epidemiology of sexual boundary violations has some variation – what is your working view about how widespread an issue this is in the psychological therapies?*

GG The simple answer is that we don't know the prevalence (Gabbard and Lester 1995). There are questionnaire surveys, but they all have notorious methodological problems. The return rate is low. Those who fill out the questionnaire may be different than those who don't complete the survey. Many do not trust the confidentiality of their responses since there is often numerical coding involved. Some people don't tell the truth on questionnaire surveys. We certainly cannot rely on figures from ethics committees and licensing boards because they see only the tip of the iceberg. What I can say from over 30 years of evaluating and treating practitioners with boundary violations is that it is not rare.

JC *You have led the way in enabling a conversation about boundary-less professionals to take place internationally, yet there remains significant and sometimes virulent denial of the extent of the problem in some quarters – do you have a view about why you think this is?*

GG Sexual boundary violations are quite close to the incest situation symbolically. Someone in authority who should care about you and protect you instead exploits you for his/her own sexual pleasure. It taps something in all of us that is abhorrent, but unconsciously desired. There is a line in Sophocles' *Oedipus Rex*, where the chorus, commenting on Oedipus, says something to the effect of: "He did what most men only dream of." There is a huge tendency to project this vulnerability into a handful of psychopaths rather than to acknowledge the universal vulnerability, that is, it is an occupational hazard for all of us. One of the things I've noticed is that often when these boundary violations come out, there's been knowledge in the practitioner community, but nobody really wanted to say. It's like they see it but they don't see it. One of the things that goes on in these cases is this: often the community of practitioners have a secret admiration for this guy who gets away with things. That makes it difficult sometimes to get information from the community because no one wants to say anything. A lot of these senior practitioners are experienced, president of some organization, and respected by others. They often are good referral sources. They send patients to other people. They want to be loyal. They don't want to lose their referral source, so they say nothing.

CULTURAL IMPERATIVES

Gabbard gives an example of a practitioner claiming that he had saved a patient from suicide by having sex with her. "They look you right in the eye and they believe it. It's not just a story, it's a rationalisation that they use to depart from their usual standards, and they think you've got a problem because you don't understand this. It's amazing: "Sometimes you have to do something unorthodox to save the patient…" I've been interested in cinematic and TV depictions of psychotherapy. The audiences tend to love the kind of guy who'll do something radical to save the patient. Then in the same film the ethics committee is depicted as a group of stuffy old men who say: "You shouldn't be doing that." You know there's a huge cultural influence to be that kind of maverick who does his own thing. And that's seductive."

REFERENCES

Coe, J. (2010) *USA Responses To Professional Boundary Violations*. London: Winston Churchill Memorial Trust.

Gabbard, G.O. (1989) *Sexual Exploitation in Professional Relationships*. Washington D.C.: American Psychiatric Press.

Gabbard, G.O. and Gutheil, T.G. (1992) 'Obstacles to the dynamic understanding of therapist-patient sexual relations.' *American Journal of Psychotherapy 46*, 515–525.

Gabbard, G.O. and Lester, E. (1995) *Boundaries and Boundary Violations in Psychoanalysis*. USA: American Psychiatric Publishing.

Gabbard, G.O. and Myers, M. (2008) *The Physician as Patient*. USA: American Psychiatric Publishing.

Schoener, G.E. (1989) *Psychotherapists' Sexual Involvement with their Clients: Intervention and Prevention*. Minneapolis: Walk-In counselling Center.

Snowden, P. (2010) 'Dealing with offending doctors: sanctions and remediation.' In Subotsky, F., Bewley, S. and Crowe, M. (eds) *Abuse of the Doctor-Patient Relationship*. London: RCPsych Publications.

FURTHER READING

Gutheil, T.G. (2005) 'Boundaries, Blackmail, and Double Binds: A Pattern Observed in Malpractice Consultation.' *Journal of the American Academy of Psychiatry and the Law 33*, 4, 476–481.

Gutheil, T.G. and Gabbard, G.O. (1993) The concept of boundaries in clinical practice: theoretical and risk management dimensions. *American Journal of Psychiatry 150*, 188–196.

Richardson, S. (2008) *Broken Boundaries: Stories of Betrayal in Relationships of Care*. London: Witness.

Subotsky, F., Bewley, S. and Crowe, M. (eds) (2010) *Abuse of the Doctor-Patient Relationship*. London: RCPsych Publications.

Chapter 4

THERAPY IN PERVERSITY: SEDUCTION, DESTRUCTION AND KEEPING BALANCE

David Jones

Overview

This chapter considers sexual offending, its relationship to healthy sexuality, the cultural slipperiness of such terms and the nature of extreme boundary violations with their complex and challenging implications for therapeutic work. While cultural and social understandings shift according to time and place, the destructiveness of perverse exploitation remains as a key reference point for therapy and therapists. Team and individual therapist dynamics require constant reflection.

INTRODUCTION

This chapter will consider sexual offending, its relationship to healthy sexuality, the cultural slipperiness of such terms and the nature of extreme boundary violations with their complex and challenging implications for therapeutic work.

Writing about people who offend sexually is fraught with difficulties. The term 'sex offender' has a wide application and the legal definition is complicated and prone to change and redefinition (Crown Prosecution Service 2010). Changes in the law seek to reflect prevailing social and political trends but they sometimes appear to run counter to other powerful cultural changes. For example, the twentieth century brought an awareness of sexuality in infants and children, the dissolution of the myth of female 'purity' (Freedman 1987) and the relaxation of many sexual constraints and prohibitions. The consequent changes in boundaries affected social, commercial and personal worlds (Hoffman 2005). At the same time there emerged a much greater awareness of the extent of sexual abuse of children, paedophilia, rape and other sexual violence (Davies 1998). Furthermore, the legal framework differs from jurisdiction to jurisdiction and some of these major social and legal changes occurred in some parts of the world but not in others. For example, the removal of legal sanction against sexual acts between members of the same gender is not universal (Bhatnagar 2010) and in some parts of the world such acts are treated as capital offences.

While the law struggles to keep a balance between cultural norms, individual freedoms and protecting vulnerable people, the media and a large proportion of the population often appear to have a very clear idea of what is 'wrong' and what is 'bad' in the field of sexual relations. This reflects the powerful unconscious forces that affect societies and which result in splits (polarisation) and projection onto others, who may be a good fit in any case. This is particularly germane when it relates to offences against children or violence towards women. At times the feelings engendered and the subsequent projection and projective identification can be so strong that they are used to justify serious assault or murder (BBC 2009; Jones 2004; White 2006). The same kind of disapproval can be found among some correctional staff in prisons (Higgins and Ireland 2009). This is in sharp contrast to another facet of popular culture, films and, particularly, pop videos, which frequently depict sexual violence against women, and glamorise and minimise the harm done by such acts (Bufkin and Eschholz 2000). While depictions of sexual offences against children are more unusual, the boundary between child/adult women (not available/available) is often represented in a highly ambiguous fashion.

It is these ambivalences that are split and enacted through a variety of conflicting social groupings or moral codes. Nevertheless, the facets of such splits exist, from a very early age, in the minds of all of us. It is the manner of the containment of such splits and the relationship to the internal mother/ father, sister/brother with all of its rivalries and incestuous ramifications that largely determine, through projection and projective identification (Göka, Yüksel and Göral 2006), the nature of future affectional and sexual bonds.

Curiously, and as a further illustration of 'slipperiness', there is a setting where two boundaries are crossed with little cost to the perpetrators in terms of stigma or social standing. This is in prison, where it is possible (for some) to have sex with another man and not be labelled a homosexual and for that sex to be forced without being labelled as rape, at least within the context of that social group (Human Rights Watch 2001). The mechanism of this requires the perpetrator to designate his (male) victim as a woman. This may be confirmed by the use of derogatory terms like queen, pretty girl or bitch. Furthermore, the perpetrator may justify the rape by saying that the victim secretly wanted the sexual contact, a distortion commonly used following incidents of sexual offence against women (Scully and Marolla 1985). A perpetrator may well have his position and status enhanced and be 'served' by the surrogate 'woman' for many years. This phenomenon is in part explained by the suggestion that actually many men have fantasies of rape and would rape if they could feel certain that they would not be caught (Scully and Marolla 1985). As one patient said to me while describing the frenetic nature and wide variety of his sexual encounters:

Fucking…, it doesn't matter who, or what, it is, it's all in the mind.

What all this delineates is an uncertainty about boundaries, a notion that time or cultural setting can impinge upon what is allowable. It suggests a conflict between basic human drives and socially constructed relationships. Such an idea is not new, of course, and was described by Freud in the *Three Essays on the Theory of Sexuality* (Freud 1991). The polymorphous sexuality of the human infant retains its place as a component in the internal world going through stages of development or, perhaps more accurately, containment. However, the unbridled demand for sensual satisfaction permitted to the infant or the vigorous expression of sexuality of the adolescent become unsatisfactory for adult relationships and social living, but only in so far as permissions change (Gordon 2008). It is not the act itself that constitutes the infraction but the absence of consent, the meaning of the offending act within the social context and the act as representative of a state of mind. In psychodynamic terms it is where the individual sits on the continua along the three axes, adult (whole object) ↔ infantile (part object), libidinal (life giving) ↔ destructive impulses, and good ↔ bad parts of the self (Sanders 1993), which determines the range and degree of perverse sexual impulses (Lubbe 2008).

Perversity seeks to turn good into bad, love into hatred and revenge, and creative sexual intercourse into the theft of pleasure. The 'slipperiness' of these concepts brings their own difficulties, for therapists, particularly as they relate to an ethical framework which may be more complex than in the treatment of other offenders (Adshead and Mezey 1993). There may often be an element of coercion in therapeutic work, the spoken or unspoken suggestion that work has to be done before release. There are specific expectations regarding confidentiality, risk and public protection and, indeed, the work may be defined as done in the interest of the 'public' instead of, or as well as, the patient (Glaser 2010).

WIDESPREAD NATURE OF SEXUAL ABUSE

Sexual abuse is widespread and presents in multifarious guises. Research has been easier to conduct with some captive and compliant/coerced offenders. Most are men and many, but not all, have been sexually abused themselves. There are others who are never held responsible for their acts or whose acts seem so far beyond the usual social limits they do not present for treatment or achieve a successful treatment result. In her book *How Could She?*, Dana Fowley describes the years of sexual abuse that she and her sister experienced from her mother, stepfather, grandparents and numerous acquaintances (Fowley 2010). As the title suggests, it is difficult to understand how a mother can herself be so abusive and, in addition, complicit in arranging for others to abuse her daughters. It is less difficult when one becomes aware of the cycle of abuse within a community where boundaries have been beaten down by the pressure of unmediated self-indulgence and where there is an absence of love. In a rare study, consisting of 40 offenders, Faller found that such women were usually impoverished, with limited education, along with marked difficulties in psychological and social functioning. About half had mental health problems, including learning difficulties and psychotic illness (Faller 1987). This is in marked contrast to the hundreds of men, in over twenty countries, who, as priests, used the Catholic Church as a vehicle to obtain sexual gratification through the abuse of children, or the men who incorporated a paedophile ring into the child care system in Islington Borough Council. This included a man who had become Director of Social Work Education at the National Institute for Social Work and who was later convicted of importing paedophilic literature (Davies 1998). These were educated men who were often in positions of power and privilege with the opportunity to consider, formulate and discuss their interests and their actions at a sophisticated level. These men may often have justified their abuses as acts of love. However, the likelihood is that the ambiguity, confusion and guilt created in the minds of their victims would be more damaging than a more clearly aggressive and singular act when responsibility is more clear (Briggs and Hawkins 1996).

Human sexuality finds expression in many varied ways. Because most of these acts are capable of possessing benign and/or malign properties, an offence can be thought of as being caused by something within the social context and within the minds of the perpetrator and the victim rather than the nature of the act itself. An offence constitutes a breach of trust and the crossing of personal boundaries which exist in the mind at the time of the offence. Although this is essentially a subjective position, it is nevertheless possible to describe the parameters of healthy sexuality, albeit in an aspirational way, as being non-coercive, with consent given by partners of equal power and being an activity which enriches the lives of participants.

BOUNDARY VIOLATIONS AND SEXUALITY: KEEPING THERAPEUTIC BALANCE

There are few areas of psychotherapeutic work where an understanding of personal, social and legal boundaries is as important as in the field of sexuality and sexual abuse. The descriptions of experience, whether with victim or perpetrator, will almost certainly extend beyond the personal experience of the therapist and may well evoke feelings of great intensity. Previous work has shown how psychotherapists, when presented with material related to an immature and unintegrated part of their own personality, can act out through denial, rejection or worse. This was particularly apparent in the attitude of many psychoanalysts to homosexual patients and candidates for training until quite recently (Jones 2001).

The therapeutic work can be very confusing. A patient once said to me, 'Did you never go straight up to a girl you didn't know and kiss her?' This apparently innocuous question was actually one by which the patient invited me, as a therapist, into a collusive relationship, a perversion of the transference which could quickly have become irredeemable. The offences that this man had committed involved inviting prostitutes to a hotel room on the basis of straight sexual intercourse, tying them up, gagging them, beating them and committing other acts of sexual invasion against their will. His remark was an illustration of the way that perverse sexuality repeats in the patterns of everyday life and in the therapeutic encounter. It becomes a form of parallel offending.

Such transgressions may be subtle and a therapist may be drawn into a perverse therapeutic relationship which may or may not give the appearance of progression but which really becomes a kind of hideout where the patient can gain support for the repetition of his activities (Meltzer 1979). The danger for the therapist is that, oblivious to the way they have been drawn into a web, they may over-identify with the victim within the patient and lose sight of the risk they present. They may feel driven to protect the patient against colleagues who 'do not understand' and they may become defensive when asked about this. Such situations can pose a serious risk within teams, creating splits which appear to be between 'punitive' and 'therapeutic' camps but which more accurately should be seen as the enactment of the split transference/ counter-transference. The harsh superego (disapproving parental object) and the deprived, maltreated, infant object will be encapsulated to such an extent that projection occurs not just onto but into others, fostering acting out within teams. While the long-term objective may be to assist the patient in integrating these split parts of the mind to create a coherent ego structure, the danger for the individual therapist and the team is that the split projections come to reside in different individuals or professional groups. This carries the risk that the therapist may experience a counter-transference which is seriously unbalanced, while the team may become dangerously split, argue, become unable to discuss key therapeutic issues and lose sight of the risks they are required to address.

So important is this matter of perversion of the transference that it is best to be forewarned and to self-consciously take structural steps to minimise the risk of catastrophic acting out and other boundary breaches. The first step is to recognise that the danger applies to all members of staff irrespective of seniority or experience. Whereas junior or new staff may receive good levels of support, supervision and oversight, this changes for more senior staff who can believe that they are protected by age and experience. It is all too easy for any therapist working closely with perverse patients to fall into a narcissistic delusion that our skill and awareness can engage and resolve a complex dynamic; or in another variation, to over-invest in the destructive pseudo-infant part of the patient and attempt to save him. Working with perverse patients when sexual boundary breaches are a constituent part of the psychopathology requires an absence of professional pride, and teams should seek to develop an open culture possibly using tools such as Interpersonal Dynamics (Reiss and Kirtchuk 2009) or a refinement, the Interface of Meaning and Projective Formulation (impF) (Babb and Canning 2011). These approaches require the involvement of the multi-disciplinary team and seek to enable and structure team thinking so that the nuances of the transference and counter-transference relations can be captured, understood and worked with.

ASSESSMENT AND MANAGEMENT OF RISK

The previous section suggests that there is an ever-present risk of boundary violation and that procedures relating to support, supervision and team-working should be established. This section considers how to assess the risk of future offending.

Given the 'slipperiness', the confusion and the perverse dynamics that exist in relation to sexual offending, a multi-dimensional approach may provide the richest understanding. In addition to monitoring transference and counter-transference processes, the Hare Psychopathy Checklist, Revised (PCL-R) and the Historical, Clinical, Risk 20 (HCR-20) can provide a firm baseline against which other findings may be compared. If a patient who scores high on the PCL-R, for example, appears to make substantial improvement within a relatively short time span, then careful attention should be given to the possibility of a collusive transference.

The psychological concept of cognitive distortions is widely used, although on its own it is really insufficiently detailed and too rigid for clinical use. Recent work has elucidated causal theories underlying such distortions, thus creating possibilities for a more dynamic understanding (Ward 2000). Developing this idea further, Beech, Fisher and Ward (2005) concluded that sexual murderers and other violent sexual offenders share five core beliefs:

- Women are unknowable (dangerous)
- Dangerous world
- Male sex drive is uncontrollable
- Entitlement
- Women as sexual objects.

Each of these can be understood in terms of perverse, pre-oedipal object relations and contextualised within Meltzer's (1979) three-dimensional formulation of sexuality. The dynamic model can be applied individually according to the pattern of relationships established by the patient in his offending and other interactions. This enables the fine grain of personality structure to be perceived in terms of risk according to the individual's current position on the three axes, as described above (Meltzer 1979, p.67; Sanders 1993, p.55; Stein 2004):

- adult (whole object) ↔ infantile (part object)
- libidinal (life giving) ↔ destructive impulses
- good ↔ bad parts of the self.

Thus, for example, each of these areas can be assessed in terms of the maturity and integrity of the personality structure, the predominance of destructiveness and the balance of good and bad parts of the self in the make-up of the personality. The first two of these represent dynamic features which may fluctuate, sometimes quite rapidly. The third, good and bad parts of the self, refers to more or less stable parts of the personality formed by processes of projection and introjection over many years. This is a simplified account of complex ideas which are described more fully elsewhere (Sanders 1993; Spillius 1983).

Women are unknowable (dangerous). While the core belief may be that 'women are seen as inherently different from men and that these differences cannot be readily understood by men', in the mind of the offender the hostile breast (maternal object) dominates the nurturing breast, leaving the ego structure alienated and threatened. Understanding is limited and attempts to understand are attacked. The hostile breast is felt to be all-knowing and lecherously exploitative.

Dangerous world. 'The offender sees the world as a dangerous place and believes that other people are likely to behave in an abusive and rejecting manner to promote their own interests. Therefore, it is necessary to fight back or fight first and achieve dominance and control over other people.' In the mind there is an excess of destructiveness and bad objects. Relief is sought by projecting the destructiveness out onto others, but little real relief is found since the external world becomes ever more threatening in a vicious cycle.

Male sex drive is uncontrollable. 'Men's sexual energy is difficult to control and women have a key role in its loss of control.' This belief may arise from the demands of the destructive and uncontained infant/pseudo-infant. It operates in relation to the denigrated female object who should know and understand the needs of the uncontrollable infant. Obstruction to these demands can be felt as deliberate and sly.

Entitlement. 'Because of their superior status such individuals feel they have the right to assert their needs above others and to expect that this will be acknowledged and agreed to by those who are judged to be less important.' This arises from grandiose feelings related to the domination of destructive impulses and unrestrained infantile greed over creative sexuality. This represents a high degree of destructive narcissism seeking to own and control the maternal object.

Women as sexual objects. 'Offenders see women existing in a constant state of sexual reception and believe that they have been created to meet the sexual needs of men.' The patient experiences women as 'existing in a constant state of sexual arousal and desire, even if they do not know it.' This belief mainly arises from destructive narcissism and intrusive identification with the sexualised maternal object. A part of the patient is projected into the mother (victim), taking up residence in the genital/anal area of the phantasy body. The aim of the projection is to exercise omnipotent control over the woman, who is in any case willing despite what she may say.

CONCLUSION

The issue of sexual offending as boundary breach has been considered in this chapter. The 'slippery' nature of the concepts as well as the social and the legal rules have been illustrated. While physical acts are clearly central to offending, it is suggested that it is the state of mind that dictates the severity of the psychological injury and that this is dependent upon consents, expectations and power together with the dynamic status of the internal world. When working with such offender patients it is important to be aware of perverse transferences and wherever possible seek confirmation from colleagues and supervisors. Team-working can be protective.

Sexual acts, and their psychological equivalent, can be in the service of love or the service of hate depending upon the balance of destructiveness and the maturity of the object relations involved. The level of risk can be judged in psychodynamic terms using a three-axis model, adult (whole object) ↔ infantile (part object), libidinal (life giving) ↔ destructive impulses and good ↔ bad parts of the self (Sanders 1993), supported by psychometric instruments such as the PCL-R and HCR-20.

REFERENCES

Adshead, G. and Mezey, G. (1993) 'Ethical issues in the psychotherapeutic treatment of paedophiles: Whose side are you on?' *Journal of Forensic Psychiatry 4*, 2, 361.

Babb, R.S. and Canning, J. (2011) 'Interface of Meaning and Projection Formulation: A Reflective Practice Tool for the Multidisciplinary Team who Works with Personality Disordered Offenders.' *Introducing the Interface of Meaning and Projection Formulation.* Available at http://impf.co.uk, accessed on 23 February 2012.

BBC (2009) 'Victim was "mistaken paedophile".' *BBC.* Available at http://news.bbc.co.uk/1/hi/england/lancashire/8255858.stm, accessed on 23 February 2012.

Beech, A., Fisher, D. and Ward, T. (2005) 'Sexual Murderers' Implicit Theories.' *Journal of Interpersonal Violence 20*, 11, 1366–1389.

Bhatnagar, A. (2010) 'Homosexuality and Society: An Insight into the Violation of the Rights of the Homosexuals and the Role of Law.' *SSRN eLibrary.* Available at http://papers.ssrn.com/sol3/papers.cfm?abstract_id=1663281, accessed on 23 February 2012.

Briggs, F. and Hawkins R. (1996) 'A comparison of the childhood experiences of convicted male child molesters and men who were sexually abused in childhood and claimed to be nonoffenders.' *Journal of Child Abuse and Neglect 20*, 3, 221–233.

Bufkin, J. and Eschholz, S. (2000) 'Images of Sex and Rape.' *Violence Against Women 6*, 12, 1317–1344.

Crown Prosecution Service (2010) *Sexual Offences Act: Legal Guidance.* The Crown Prosecution Service.

Davies, N. (1998) 'The sheer scale of child sexual abuse in Britain.' Available at www.nickdavies.net/1998/04/01/the-sheer-scale-of-child-sexual-abuse-in-britain, accessed on 23 February 2012.

Faller, K.C. (1987) 'Women who sexually abuse children.' *Violence and Victims 2*, 4, 263–276.

Fowley, D. (2010) *How Could She?* London: Arrow, Random House.

Freedman, E.B. (1987) '"Uncontrolled Desires": The Response to the Sexual Psychopath 1920–1960.' *The Journal of American History 74*, 1, 83–106.

Freud, S. (1991) *On Sexuality: Three Essays on the Theory of Sexuality and Other Works* (New edition). London: Penguin Books.

Glaser, B. (2010) 'Sex offender programmes: New technology coping with old ethics.' *Journal of Sexual Aggression: An international, interdisciplinary forum for research, theory and practice 16*, 3, 261.

Göka, E., Yüksel, F.V. and Göral, F.S. (2006) 'Projective identification in human relations.' *Türkpsikiyatridergisi, Turkish Journal of Psychiatry 17*, 1, 46.

Gordon, H. (2008) 'The treatment of paraphilias: An historical perspective.' *Criminal Behaviour and Mental Health 18*, 2, 79–87.

Higgins, C. and Ireland, C.A. (2009) 'Attitudes towards male and female sex offenders: a comparison of forensic staff, prison officers and the general public in Northern Ireland.' *British Journal of Forensic Practice 11*, 1, 14–19.

Hoffman, L. (2005) 'Freud's Theories About Sex As Relevant as Ever.' *Psychiatric News 40*, 15, 18.

Human Rights Watch (2001) *No Escape: Male Rape in U.S. Prisons*. Human Rights Watch.

Jones, D. (2001) 'Shame, Disgust, Anger and Revenge: Homosexuality and Countertransference.' *British Journal of Psychotherapy 17*, 4, 493–504.

Jones, D. (2004) 'Murder as an attempt to manage self disgust.' In D. Jones (ed.) *Working with Dangerous People: The Psychotherapy of Violence*. Oxford: Radcliffe Publishing.

Lubbe, T. (2008) 'A Kleinian Theory of Sexuality.' *British Journal of Psychotherapy 24*, 3, 299–316.

Meltzer, D. (1979) *Sexual States of Mind*. London: Karnac Books.

Reiss, D. and Kirtchuk, G. (2009) 'Interpersonal dynamics and multidisciplinary teamwork.' *Journal of Advanced Psychiatric Treatment 15*, 6, 462–469.

Sanders, K. (1993) 'The Economics of Introjective Identification and the Embarrassment of Riches.' *British Journal of Psychotherapy 10*, 2, 136–141.

Scully, D. and Marolla, J. (1985) '"Riding the Bull at Gilley's": Convicted Rapists Describe the Rewards of Rape.' *Social Problems 32*, 3, 251–263.

Spillius, E.B. (1983) 'Some Developments from the Work of Melanie Klein.' *International Journal of Psycho-Analysis 64*, 321–332.

Stein, A. (2004) 'Fantasy, Fusion, And Sexual Homicide.' *Contemporary Psychoanalysis 40*, 495–517.

Ward, T. (2000) 'Sexual offenders' cognitive distortions as implicit theories.' *Aggression and Violent Behaviour 5*, 5, 491–507.

White, D. (2006) 'Loving the Alien: A Moral Re-Evaluation of Paedophiles.' In S.N. Fhlainn (ed.) (2008) *Dark Reflections, Monstrous Reflections: Essays on the Monster in Culture*. Oxford: Inter-Disciplinary Press. Available at www.inter-disciplinary.net/publishing-files/idp/eBooks/drmr%201.3c.pdf, accessed on 23 February 2012.

Chapter 5

GROUPWORK FOR OFFENCE PERPETRATORS WITH A HISTORY OF BOUNDARY VIOLATION IN THE HOSPITAL SETTING

Estelle Moore and Emma Ramsden[1]

It is the awareness of how stuck you are that makes you recover.

Anon

Overview

- When damage has already been done, and even repeated within hospital services, how might we work hopefully with the subject of boundary?

- Describing the service users, facilitators, groupwork approach and presence of clinical consultancy supervision.

- Suggestions for creative methods for addressing the subject of boundaries in groups.

- Some examples from clinical practice.

- Concluding comments.

1   We would like to thank our colleagues Brian Thomas, Alison Dudley, Emma MacIntosh, Martha Ferrito, Darren Lumbard, Claire Wilson, Sydney Klugman and Mario Guarnieri, and group members over the years in high security, for the part they have played in enriching the ideas presented in this chapter.

INTRODUCTION

This chapter acknowledges the deep impact of abuse of boundary (in a range of forms from interpersonal violence to illicit sexual encounters), its multiple inter-generational impact via connections to further offending, and its implications for those detained for treatment within the overall context of forensic clinical services. In writing it, we attempted to hold in mind the experience of those who actively participate in treatment, facilitators of this work and the perspective of supervisors, all of whom play a part in the overall endeavour. Our focus is on groupwork as an intervention offered from a base within the Centralised Groupwork Service (CGS) at Broadmoor Hospital, a High Secure Hospital, part of the National Health Service (NHS) resource for the United Kingdom. We mention the CGS (Perkins, Moore and Dudley 2007) as a clinical service only to provide the context for our practice. High security environments have been described by others writing about psychotherapeutic work as the 'ultimate container', from which escape is almost impossible, and wherein work of considerable emotional intensity is undertaken 'safely' (Morris 2001; Gordon, Beckley and Lowings 2011).

Drawing on brief vignettes from clinical histories and completed groupwork which focus on one of the many key themes in the CGS work, family and relationship narratives, we seek to share some ideas for clinical use by staff/facilitators working with service users who have encountered and perpetrated serious and, in particular, sexual boundary violations. In the context of this work, groupwork facilitators are multi-disciplinary clinicians, who have extensive experience and specialist knowledge of working with forensic service users/group members. Confidentiality has been maintained in the compilation of this chapter with respect to both service users/group members and staff engaged in the treatment service. The clinical vignettes are composites of many events and stories that have been shared and reflected on in over a decade of groupwork.

We propose that groups, whilst inherently challenging for anyone with a history of breaches of trust, can also provide a manageable forum to explore interpersonal conflicts and actions without 'over-stimulating' arousal. We proceed with great care in cases where abuse occurred with an audience, and where the echoes of previous betrayals in platonic or/and sexually intimate (1:1) encounters remain unresolved. With the potential value of group interventions as our starting position, we have devised, adapted and developed a range of techniques and ideas for holding boundaries in mind. These aim to embolden clinical effectiveness via the inclusion, alongside verbal discussion, of creative and action-based methods that support the process of boundary maintenance. Opportunities are thus elicited which invite all service users/group members to make a contribution to self-knowledge and gain shared understanding in this area. The internal concept of trust has in itself a complex range of embedded boundaries which employ, provide and nurture safety towards self and others. Trust requires communication, collaboration, support and engagement and its presence is a core and vital aspect of being in any group. The transition from being perceived as 'untrustworthy' to 'trusted' is emerging as a key shift in identity and therefore a marker of change for those who have resided in a high security hospital (Tapp 2011).

In this chapter we outline example techniques, such as the 'timeline' and 'containers', alongside experiences of engagement with group members and reflect on their use via clinical vignettes. Further, a narrative is offered around the provision of consultancy clinical supervision, a key element of clinical practice, in which significant experience of the client field is equally held by both supervisors and practitioners (Hawkins and Shohet 2002). Paying attention to staff needs, roles and responsibilities is a key element in any therapeutic approach or model (e.g. Hamilton 2010; Talkes and Tennant 2004). Clinical supervision is integral to ensuring the onward safety of clinical practice, as it provides boundaries, such as time and continuity (Sheets 2000). Supervision supports the clinical process so that group members can develop, through meaningful reflection of emergent themes, their understanding of key events and experiences (Jones 1996). Good clinical practice is based on considerations of interrelationship dynamics as well as thematic focus, treatment goals, outcome measures, and formative, summative and longitudinal evaluations of behaviour, action and intention (Horvath and Symonds 1991; Norcross 2002). Not to acknowledge the impact of witnessing or encountering trauma, even through stories and re-telling, would compromise safety by increasing the vulnerability of staff to unhelpful responses to complex material or encounters with (already traumatised) individuals.

The groupwork service engages clinical supervisors who are in the main internal clinicians within the hospital. All have significant clinical experience in the field as facilitators and supervisors and some have undertaken formal postgraduate training in clinical supervision. It is therefore often the case that the clinical supervisors and facilitators will be known colleagues and inevitably these professional alliances add their own set of dynamics to the groupwork task.

VIOLATIONS OF BOUNDARY WITHIN MENTAL HEALTH SERVICES: TAKING UP THE ISSUES IN TREATMENT

Violation of a boundary in a forensic mental health service is as serious as it sounds: it can implicate staff and service users in a process which falls outside all that is 'normal', 'professional' and 'therapeutic' simultaneously. Given that the key objective of staff in forensic services is the provision of *safety* and the *protection of others* (and self), boundary violations generate heightened anxiety at every level of the organisation, with an increased potential for unconsciously 'acting-out' activity to occur. How best to work with those who live in hospital with a history of involvement in boundary violations has been an enduring question for therapy services for some time. Inevitably, to understand events in the present, information from the past is highly relevant. Re-viewing events in the presence of new witnesses (the others in the group, including staff) can be made tolerable via exercises which provide a supportive framework or 'scaffolding' process in the direction of resilience.

It could be argued that all therapeutic groupwork is concerned with operating safely and within recognised, professional and regulated boundaries, and reinforcing or repeatedly rehearsing their importance. This will take place via session content in all the groups that address offending specifically (e.g. in groupwork on violence and sexual offending). We also offer specific sessions to educate, focus and explore the subject of boundary and the impact of past violation: understanding relationships and intimacy (URI) is a themed group, for example, with specific targets to examine closeness and distance in encounters with others.

Groups are widely offered within NHS settings and forensic settings in particular (Tschuschke and Dies 1994): every group generates a unique psychological climate which provides the basis for therapeutic factors to operate. As in other therapies, groups require a positive working alliance to be established among the facilitators, between facilitators and group members, and in group members with each other (Thomas-Peter and Garrett 2000). Alliances are formed regardless of the theme or focus of the group, and facilitators critically reflect upon these throughout all stages of the group's life, both in the forum of the group itself and in clinical supervision (Gardner and Coombs 2010).

LINKING PAST AND PRESENT: UNDERMINING THE IMPACT OF TRAUMA

Physical and sexual abuse, parental neglect, poverty, criminality, family breakdown and placement outside the home of origin are features of life which have directly impacted on the development of the majority of those referred to high security forensic services (Taylor 1997). It is well known that the brain and its capacity to process information (Bennouna-Greene *et al.* 2011) is affected by maltreatment (de Zulueta 2006; Wilkinson 2006), and that clinical sequelae may stem in part from enduring and adverse effects on brain development (Andersen *et al.* 2008). Felson and Lane (2009) analysed data from inmates in State and Federal Correctional Facilities in the United States, and reported that offenders model specific behaviours to which they have been exposed. They explore the literature on 'specialisation' (i.e. offences with a unique aetiology) and find some evidence for social learning theory, whereby, for example, violent offenders are much more likely to engage in additional violent offences than their non-violent counterparts; sexual offenders show some tendency to specialise in sexual crime 'against a backdrop of much versatility' (Lussier 2005, p.288).

What might such research mean for the task of intervention, and in particular with service users/group members when their interpersonal boundaries have been broken in health care settings? Felson and Lane (2009) argue for the application of social learning theory: abuse produces a hostility bias, which in turn is associated with patterns of violence consistent with post-traumatic stress. This research team highlights the importance of knowing what children have learnt from their encounters and observations of an abusive model, in order to assist in understanding why they might have replicated actions in the future.

For therapists seeking to promote change and the inhibition of maladaptive patterns in such a complex area, a major goal, regardless of therapeutic orientation, is to search for and unpack themes in what might have been learnt, and to explore alternative responses to this (Quayle and Moore 2006). This process occurs in a myriad ways in forensic focused sessions and services (e.g. Dowdswell, Akerman and Lawrence 2010; Hollin 2006; McGuire 2008). Functional analytic approaches clarify for offenders the factors that contribute to the development, expression and maintenance of presenting problems such as aggression (Daffern and Howells 2009). In group treatment, starting work on this might be operationalised via the use of a 'timeline' (described below). This task explores connections between events in life, thoughts, actions and internalised messages and meanings, and can comprise whole modules or phases of interventions, including groupwork with violent and sexual offenders, where histories are highly complex and reduction in future risk is the primary objective.

EXPLORATION OF BOUNDARIES: WITH 'FAMILY' AND 'RELATIONSHIPS' IN MIND

The theme of 'family' is one which inevitably arises in many aspects of psychological treatment for those with long-standing and complex presentations. A 'Family Awareness' group has been offered at Broadmoor Hospital in various forms over the last 20 years (Moore *et al.* 2000; Quayle,

France and Wilkinson 1996); similarly, interpersonal relationships have been explored to address intimacy difficulties often associated with sexual offending (Quayle and Moore 2006). Groups such as these endure as treatment options because they attempt to work with those whose recollections of trauma and conflict with 'family' remain unresolved. The lack of resolution provides the context for the genesis of offending motives, action and chronic loneliness.

We all come from a family, so for the facilitator to be part of a group looking at family re-creates a family group at some level. Each person sits with their knowledge of their childhood journey, their sibling or only-child relationships, and the canon of roles within their family (e.g. mother, brother, child, carer, father, youngest, eldest, cousin, aunt, uncle). Therefore, all of the associated boundaries (and, for some, memories of their violation) are present in this exchange, alongside the social and functional roles of group members. Hierarchies relating to age, and time spent in incarcerated settings, offending and in hospital are all relevant. For staff, issues such as their gender, pay grade and clinical responsibility in relation to other facilitators, service provision, research and development, knowledge and alliance with service users/group members prior to the group's commencement, and then the dynamics within the group's developing process, will be relevant.

ACTION-BASED METHODS: ADDRESSING THE SUBJECT OF BOUNDARIES IN GROUPS

Techniques developed within this groupwork are drawn from an eclectic range of arts-based, social and psychological resources, influenced by facilitators' experiences, publications and other literature from a range of client settings. These focus on topics such as working with offenders in practice, self-awareness, interrelatedness and affect management (Barker 1989; Boal 1979; Holland and Ward 1990; Spolin 1998; Sunderland and Engleheart 1993).

The inclusion of social skills and drama processes like role play and problem solving in pairs and teams presents opportunities for rehearsal of the presence, or absence, of limits that protect (Gutheil 2005). Also, individual methods like projective techniques which incorporate working with small objects to create images, and story-making using art processes, communicate feelings via abstractions, metaphor and symbol (Jones 1996; Lahad 2000). Musical opportunities can be offered as an alternative communication tool for expression of mood, temperament, pace or emotional flow.

Any of these methods may also be utilised in the supervisory space. Sand trays and small objects, a comprehensive range of creative picture cards such as the 'blob people' and the 'bears' (see resource details), which depict both group dynamics and emotional states, can facilitate a creative reflection on groupwork process and focus on individual exchanges.

Group members are invited to engage with action-based exercises at various points throughout the different stages of the group's life: at the outset, during the established stage, and in the process of ending. Examples from all three stages are outlined below. It is intended within these invitations to engage in explorations other than sitting and talking, develop further existing interpersonal skills, and encounter new experiences. These experiences enable the concept of boundary to be explored and played with safely, by engaging both physical body and mind. By asking group members to step outside of their usual experience, the intention is to offer a new paradigm for relating and to encounter the emergent group's themes by engagement in a multi-layered approach. The groupwork process, like any therapeutic space, is an opportunity to try out new skills and take (safe) risks with historically fragile and vulnerable identities.

Early stage: Timeline exercise

This is a task in which group members are invited to create a living document, which is developed throughout the group's life, that charts events of significance in their history. A mixture of drawing and writing using arts materials can be offered to complete the task. Timelines are presented back to the group, and authors can then be 'hot-seated', which denotes being asked questions by other group members and facilitators in order to expand events charted and gain a richer understanding of them.

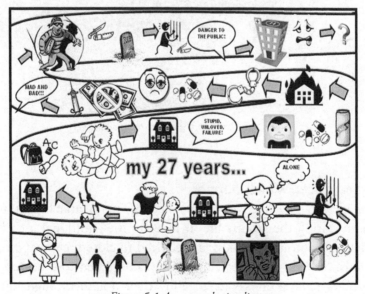

Figure 5.1 An example timeline

Established stage: Containers exercise

This exercise aims to elicit awareness and understanding of personal boundaries. A series of empty containers are presented on a table or in the middle of the group's circle. The containers are different sizes, shapes and textures, and have a range of competency to contain physical matter. Containers are drawn from eclectic environments, including work and home (safety permitting in forensic settings). A typical array of boxes for this exercise may contain a glasses case, a Tupperware box, a decorative box for holding potpourri or similar, a baking jar (maybe slightly broken or missing a lid), a cardboard box, a transparent box, an ineffective box and so on. Group members are invited to choose a container which represents themselves in relationship to others – for example, (i) to the group, (ii) to their family of origin, (iii) to their ward peers and carers, (iv) to themselves in the past, present or future. The group discusses their choices and findings.

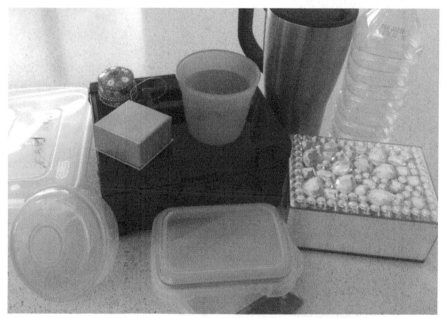

Figure 5.2 Example of a collection of containers

Established stage: Which potato?

This exercise can be effective when reflecting upon attachment to others experienced during the group's life. It involves the additional use of trust in the facilitators as group members are required to close their eyes on a couple of occasions. Seated, with eyes closed, they are guided to a bag of potatoes and invited to choose one. After meeting their potato through touch, they replace it in the bag before opening their eyes and identifying their potato using sight first, then touch, from a range of potatoes on a table in front of them. The process is discussed as it unfolds and facilitator questions asked of group members about the nature of their attachment to their potato and ability to identify it from a range of other similar potatoes.

Established or closing stage: Desert Island
Discs (Relationship review)

The invitation to explore relationships is offered a few weeks ahead of the exercise taking place. This enables the group members to spend time away from the group, reflecting on the significant relationships in their lives, identifying music which in some way embodies the dominant themes of these relationships, and thinking how to introduce the music and the relationship to their fellow group members. Based on the format of the Radio 4 programme *Desert Island Discs*, group members are then 'interviewed' by a nominated facilitator in front of other group members and their choices of music played.

SOME CLINICAL VIGNETTES

The following clinical vignettes aim to support the chapter's theme that work through trust on boundaries is potentially beneficial if safely conducted and reflected upon. The vignettes are provided with a brief group member 'his-story' in order to contextualise the background of the individual engaging with the group process.

Whilst these exercises have developed over time in relation to the themes of boundary violations, as one of the following vignettes illustrates, within this complex population, for some service users/group members therapy can be experienced as overpowering, leading to withdrawal from it. The experience may represent many themes, among them a possible mirroring of early life experiences or boundary violations, a sustained inability to engage with an emotional understanding about safe boundary setting, a fear of change and a fear of being with others. For some, the replaying of the experience of harm in encounters with others is such that no new thinking or engagement with an inner creativity can be tolerated. This inhibits entry into an arena where new (safer) boundaries may develop.

Vignette one

The following commentary represents a very small segment of a long history of care, and a failure to engage a group member with the task of embarking on sharing something of his life history via the timeline.

His-story: Dan

Dan has a history of parental neglect from birth and from around the age of three had been witness to near-fatal domestic violence which endured intermittently but throughout his formative years. He committed a rape and murderous assault of a young female when he was aged 15. In over ten years of treatment, he had disclosed a sexually abusive experience as a boy but had never named the perpetrator. He referred to his mother as an alcoholic, with much disdain, and he refused any contact with her for long periods. In the hospital, he had been involved in more than one encounter with female nursing staff whereby he had engaged them in acts of security and sexual boundary violations and presented a number of claims that he was 'in a relationship' with them.

Dan's reaction to the invitation to 'warm-up' and generate a timeline

Dan was highly suspicious of the group and the motives of the facilitators. On entering the room he would position his chair so that he was outside the group (and the line of sight of the security cameras outside the building). He refused to engage with movement-related tasks, even when included by other group members, whilst still seated. When invited to share something of his relationships through commentary on his timeline, he closed down all questions from the group with comments implying his rejection of ideas. Quickly, and on more than one occasion, the group was silenced, and could not think of ways to include him that he might find tolerable. Events on the ward subsequently prevented him from attending the group: the experience of being 'lost' to therapeutic options was (once again) re-enacted by all.

Vignette two

This vignette illustrates the engagement of a group member referred to as Laurie with other group members, using the creative exercise 'Which potato?' The process highlighted a difficulty in making connections with the object of the exercise but not the concept or the willingness to try. It brought about connections with family life and enabled facilitators to ask meaningful questions about feelings and relationships based on the playing out of events in the exercise.

His-story: Laurie

Laurie, who always chose to sit by an open window in the group room, disclosed that his parents had never, in his recollection, shown him any warmth or concern. He was raised (e.g. taken to school, when he attended) by a half-sister only four years his senior. He recalled being shut in the airing cupboard by his mother for being 'noisy', and that 'the bottle' (alcohol) ruled their household. Both parents were dependent on alcohol. Key boundary violations that came to mind for him in the group included his witnessing of his father's sexual activities with younger men, and the connection between this and one of his offences (sexual assault). His assaults on staff in the prisons and hospitals he had resided in were physical, not sexual.

Response to the exercise   isolation of affect

Laurie was prepared to 'give anything a go', he said, and contributed without apparent concern for himself or restraint during warm-up tasks. During the potatoes exercise he was the only group member in the room who did not find his potato from amongst the others, and who could not identify it when given a second chance. He appeared crestfallen about this, but it was not possible to put these feelings into words. Fellow group members in the room demonstrated empathy: they connected to his disconnection by seeking to include him, and to give voice to his distress when he was unable to. The sense facilitators were also left with was how profound the absence of any secure attachment had been throughout his life.

Vignette three

His-story: Harry

Understanding Relationships and Intimacy group member Harry had been in hospital for more than half his life. He had sexually assaulted staff during an early part in his admission following an offence of sexual assault on a female stranger. He took up the role of 'father' figure in the group on the basis of the duration of his stay. Others tended to receive his advice warmly. The passage of time led him to reflect on the importance of equality in marital relationships: a feature missing, he felt, from what he had witnessed at home. His mother worked throughout his childhood as a sex worker based at the family home.

Response to the exercise

Harry did not disclose his history of sexual abuse (by regular client visitors of his mother) in words to the group. He chose the song 'Tears of a Clown' to illustrate his experience as a child, the words of which also carried immense poignancy for the other men in the group.

CLINICAL CONSULTANCY SUPERVISION: THE REVIEW OF PARALLEL PROCESSES TO CREATE SAFE BOUNDARIES

Some of the moments generated in groups such as this will be experienced as making a profound connection, pivoting on trust of the self and others (e.g. the group members as 'witnesses'). Experiences from the sessions are reflected on and explored during regularly scheduled supervision sessions which support the overall process. This provides a trusting and supportive forum for facilitators to review and critically reflect upon the strategies and interventions offered in groups, as well as process the feelings arising from engaging in the groupwork (Davys and Beddoe 2010; Gardner and Coombs 2010).

Reflecting on the experiences, patterns and feelings present in the staff teams enables connections to phenomena emerging within the clinical group process. Dynamics present in the facilitation team may or may not manifest in feelings raised in them by each service user's engagement, and this becomes a focus within the clinical supervision space. Connection is a universal theme relevant in all group processes, not exclusively linked to forensic histories, but mirrored in the transference relationship of facilitators' own experiences of being part of groups. How these boundaries manifest, where they relate and diverge and the potential for violation can be explored. How the boundaries articulate the position of an individual, the collective experience for the group, and perhaps both will also be relevant.

Facilitators employ skills of role modelling, introducing and negotiating safely held boundaries with group members for future safe boundaries. In turn, the facilitators are supported in the reflection of clinical material. The consultancy supervision approach engages a supervisor, often from within the staff team, who has further supervision training to accompany their existing specialised knowledge of the service user population. This interplay of experienced clinicians supports the ongoing ability for containing and working safely with boundary violations and reflections of past behaviour at a meaningful level where potential difficulty can be held and worked through.

For some supervisors in this environment, incorporating action-based and creative methods into the supervisory process has become a recognised practice. The literature suggests that their inclusion can enhance the reflective function and expand perspective-taking in the processing of clinical material (Carr and Ramsden 2008; Tselikas-Portman 1999). The potato exercise as illustrated above was experienced first in supervision and then transferred to the group. Revisiting how the group engaged with the exercise and the emergent life history was a process that returned once more to the supervisory space and led to discussions about feelings raised in the facilitator team, as well as enabling empathic reflections upon group members' experiences.

CONCLUSION

Group members in high security forensic settings have often experienced, through perpetration and victimhood, damaging and deep-rooted violations of boundaries – their own and those of others. The psychological sequelae of abuse are well established, with survivors at risk for medical, psychological, behavioural and sexual disorder (Baker, Beech and Tyson 2006; Maniglio 2009). Trauma is profound and can appear enduring if it remains unresolved, unarticulated and separate in mind from other events. To respond by hearing or witnessing stories, spoken and unspoken, in order to promote resilience, requires minute attention to detail and an attunement to need, in our view, best provided by teams of qualified staff working together.

Very few containers in life are water-tight or indestructible. They must be regularly checked and monitored to ensure that they function as they should, particularly if they are being tested for their capacity and fitness to 'retain'. Staff need a system of support to engage with such material, hold it, process it and return it with some sense of hope. To conclude, an illustration of the potential benefit, where we believe this was achieved by a 'graduate' participant from a group. He is talking here with peers about a boundary violation in which he was involved:

> No one trusts you when you are under scrutiny… My relationship with the nurse affected my family, she lost her job, her career, something she had trained for years for. It does not affect just two people, it affects lots of others. I know my boundaries now; I can take action if I think things are going in the wrong direction.

REFERENCES

Andersen, S.L., Tomadaa, A., Vincow, E.S., Valente, E., Polcari, A. and Teicher, M.H. (2008) 'Preliminary evidence for sensitive periods in the effect of childhood sexual abuse on regional brain development.' *Journal of Neuropsychiatry and Clinical Neurosciences 20*, 292–301.

Baker, E., Beech, A. and Tyson, M. (2006) 'Attachment disorganisation and sexual offending.' *Journal of Family Violence 21*, 221–231.

Barker, C. (1989) *Theatre Games, A New Approach to Drama Training.* London: Methuen.

Bennouna-Greene, V., Kremer, S., Stoetzel, C., Christmann, D. *et al.* (2011) 'Hippocampal dysgenesis and variable neuropsychiatric phenotypes in patients with Bardet-Biedl syndrome underline complex CNS impact of primary cilia.' *Clinical Genetics 80*, 6, 523–531.

Boal, A. (1979) *Theatre of the Oppressed.* London: Pluto.

Carr, M., and Ramsden, E. (2009) 'An Exploration of Supervision in Education.' In A. Davys and L. Beddoe (eds) (2010) *Best Practice in Professional Supervision.* London: Jessica Kingsley Publishers.

Daffern, M. and Howells, K. (2009). 'The function of aggression in personality disordered patients.' *Journal of Interpersonal Violence 24*, 586–600.

Davys, A. and Beddoe, L. (eds) (2010) *Best Practice in Professional Supervision.* London: Jessica Kingsley Publishers.

Desert Island Discs (2011) BBC Radio 4. 23 October 2011 at 11.15.

de Zulueta, F. (2006) *From Pain to Violence – the Traumatic Roots of Destructiveness.* Chichester: Wiley and Sons.

Dowdswell, H., Akerman, G. and Lawrence (2010) 'Unlocking offence paralleling behaviour in a custodial setting – a personal perspective from members of staff and a resident in a forensic therapeutic community.' In M. Daffern, L. Jones and J. Shine (eds) *Offence Paralleling Behaviour: A Case Formulation Approach to Offender Assessment and Intervention.* Chichester: John Wiley.

Felson, R.B. and Lane, K.J. (2009) 'Social Learning, Sexual and Physical Abuse and Adult Crime.' *Aggressive Behaviour 35*, 489–501.

Gardner, F. and Coombs, S.J. (2010) *Researching, Reflecting and Writing about Work.* London: Routledge.

Gordon, N., Beckley, K. and Lowings, G. (2011) 'Therapists' Experience of Therapy.' In P. Willmot and N. Gordon (eds) *Working Positively with Personality Disorder.* Chichester: John Wiley & Sons.

Gutheil, T.G. (2005) 'Boundary issues and personality disorders.' *Journal of Psychiatric Practice 11*, 421–429.

Hamilton L. (2010) 'The Boundary Seesaw Model: Good Fences Make for Good Neighbours.' In A. Tennant and K. Howells (eds) *Using Time, Not Doing Time: Practitioner Perspectives on Personality Disorder and Risk.* Chichester: John Wiley & Sons.

Hawkins, P. and Shohet, R. (2002) *Supervision in the Helping Professions.* Oxford: Open University Press.

Holland, S. and Ward, C. (1990) *Assertiveness: A practical approach.* Oxfordshire: Winslow Press.

Hollin, C.R. (2006) 'Offending behaviour programmes and contention: evidence-based practice, manuals and programme evaluation.' In C.R. Hollin and E.J. Palmer (eds) *Offending Behaviour Programmes: Development, Application and Controversies.* Chichester: Wiley.

Horvath, A.O. and Symonds, B.D. (1991) 'Relation between working alliance and outcome in psychotherapy. A meta-analysis.' *Journal of Counselling Psychology 38*, 139–149.

Jones, P. (1996) *Drama as Therapy – Theatre as Living.* London: Routledge.

Lahad, M. (2000) *Creative Supervision.* London: Jessica Kingsley Publishers.

Lussier, P. (2005) 'The criminal activity of sexual offenders in adulthood: Revisiting the specialisation debate.' *Sexual Abuse: A journal of research and treatment 17*, 269–292.

Maniglio, R. (2009) 'The impact of child sexual abuse on health: a systematic review of reviews.' *Clinical Psychological Review 29*, 647–657.

McGuire, J. (2008) 'A review of effective interventions for reducing aggression and violence.' *Philosophical Transactions of the Royal Society B 363*, 2577–2597.

Moore, E., Manners, A., Lee, J., Quayle, M. and Wilkinson, E. (2000) 'Trauma in the family: groupwork on family awareness for men in high security hospitals.' *Criminal Behaviour and Mental Health 10*, 242–255.

Morris, M. (2001) 'Grendon Underwood: A Psychotherapeutic Prison.' In J. Williams Saunder (ed.) *Life Within Hidden Worlds, Psychotherapy in Prisons*. London: Karnac.

Norcross, J.C. (2002) *Psychotherapy Relationships that Work: Therapist Contributions and Responsiveness to Patients*. New York, NY: Oxford University Press.

Perkins, D., Moore, E. and Dudley, A. (2007) 'Developing a Centralised Groupwork Service at Broadmoor Hospital.' *Mental Health Review Journal 12*, 1, 16–20.

Quayle, M. and Moore, E. (2006) 'Maladaptive Learning: Cognitive-Behavioural Treatment and beyond.' In C. Newrith, C. Meux and P.J. Taylor (eds) *Personality Disorder and Serious Offending. Hospital Treatment Models*. London: Hodder Arnold.

Quayle, M., France, J. and Wilkinson, E. (1996) 'An Integrated Modular Approach to Therapy in a Special Hospital Young Men's Unit.' In C. Cordess and M. Cox (eds) *Forensic Psychotherapy, Crime, Psychodynamics and the Offender Patient*. London: Jessica Kingsley Publishers.

Sheets, V.R. (2000) 'Staying in the lines.' *Nursing Management 31*, 28–34.

Spolin, V. (1998) *Improvisation for the Theatre*. Evanston, IL: Northwest University Press.

Sunderland, M. and Engleheart, P. (1993) *Draw on your Emotions*. Oxon: Winslow Press.

Talkes, K. and Tennant, A. (2004) 'The therapy seesaw: Achieving therapeutically balanced approaches to working with emotional distress.' *British Journal of Forensic Practice 6*, 3–12.

Tapp, J. (2011) 'Evaluating Change in High Security Hospital.' Unpublished PhD thesis, University of Surrey, ongoing.

Taylor, P.J. (1997) 'Damage, disease and danger.' *Criminal Behaviour and Mental Health 7*, 19–48.

Thomas-Peter, B.A. and Garrett, T. (2000) 'Preventing Sexual Contact Between Professionals and Patients in Forensic Environments.' *Journal of Forensic Psychiatry 11*, 1, 135–150.

Tschuschke, V. and Dies, R.R. (1994) 'Intensive analysis of therapeutic factors and outcome in long-term inpatient groups.' *International Journal of Group Psychotherapy 44*, 185–208.

Tselikas-Portmann, E. (ed.) (1999) *Supervision and Dramatherapy*. London: Jessica Kingsley Publishers.

Wilkinson, M. (2006) *Coming Into Mind: The mind-brain relationship: a Jungian clinical perspective*. London: Routledge.

RESOURCES

Anger Blob Cards, Speechmark Publishing Ltd, Milton Keynes, UK (www.speechmark.net)

The Bears (ISBN: 1-8756507-9-2), St Luke's Innovative Resources, Bendigo, Victoria, Australia (www.innovative resources.org)

Emotion Blob Cards, Speechmark Publishing Ltd, Milton Keynes, UK (www.speechmark.net)

Chapter 6

MOVING WITH THE PATIENT: BOUNDARY PHENOMENA IN FORENSIC DRAMATHERAPY

Mario Guarnieri

Overview

In this chapter I reflect on an aspect of my work as a dramatherapist in a high secure hospital for offenders diagnosed with mental health problems and compulsorily detained under the Mental Health Act for England and Wales. Specifically, I explore the expression of boundary phenomena as it presented in the first three years of my work with an adult male patient. I discuss it as an expression of an internal object-relating drama which seemingly could only be communicated through physically showing. I will highlight the implications of the use of the dramatherapy space itself emerging as a *potential* space in the physical, psychological and emotional interplay between the patient and the dramatherapist; through this interplay boundaries and boundariedness are discovered.

Links between dramatherapy, psychoanalytic psychotherapy, drama and theatre occur throughout the text.

INTRODUCTION

I would like to share some thoughts on my experience of the way in which boundary phenomena can be played out in the dramatherapy space, within the context of a forensic setting. Through the example of clinical material I will describe the working with and working through of a patient's verbal and especially non-verbal expressions of his internal boundary confusion. My focus will be on the significant use of the boundaried therapy space itself, with my attention being centred on the patient's impulsive physical movement within that space, and on the dramatherapist's use of his own physical associations in relation to the patient, which allows the patient to have an experience of being in a boundaried relationship to the dramatherapist.

Within the forensic setting I am referring to dramatherapy is afforded its own dedicated clinical work space. This is important given the nature of the therapy, in which physical use of the space is a significant part of the work. Therefore the physical dimensions of the therapeutic space come meaningfully into play, so that the boundaries, both physical and representational, become a critical focal point of the work.

DRAMATHERAPY AND FORENSIC SETTINGS

Many authors have linked the process of drama to what happens in the psychodynamic oriented consulting room. One example is McDougall (1986), whose thinking about her practice is contained within the metaphor of the theatre: 'Psychoanalysis is a theatre on whose stage all our psychic repertory may be played' (p.284). Further: 'In the hope of finding meaning and easing pain, two people step out on that stage to bring the drama to life as psychic reality' (p.17). McDougall is referring both to the unconscious interplay that happens in the mind within the transference and counter-transference relationship and the analytic process itself.

In dramatherapy, equal validity is given to the psychic and the physical, the internal and the external. The subject is seen in relation to the environment and in relation to the objects in that environment, which of course includes the therapist. This external relatedness gives form to the patient's psychic world and is explored as a representation of internal object-relating dramas.

Generally in the talking therapies the patient sits on a chair or lies on a couch. The patient is physically located in this spot. One of the distinctive features of dramatherapy, and poignantly so in a forensic environment, is the permission for movement and the use of objects in a concrete way, allowing the opportunity to generate a *potential* relationship to the therapeutic environment, provoking a necessary awareness of the physical boundaries: the floor, the ceiling, the walls, the door, the windows, the table, the chairs and other objects. The environment itself becomes an active part of the dramatherapy process, functioning as a potential space.

Winnicott's (1971) use of the term 'potential space' refers to an intermediate area of experiencing that lies between the inner psychic reality and actual or external reality, in the me and not-me. The forms within which this experience occurs include the play space and the psychotherapy space, as well as the areas of creativity, cultural experience and transitional phenomena (Ogden 1985). The dramatherapy space offers permission for play and creativity. However, for play and creativity (in other words for life) to flourish an individual needs to have, and to have had, confidence in the provision of a trusted and trusting environment; 'playing implies trust' (Winnicott 1971, p.51). Typically, the forensic patient has little experience of this in his or her life: 'The forensic patients' experience of their everyday environment was that it did not allow safe interaction' (Dunn Grayer 2005, p.28). The therapist's intended, benign offer of a potential space for play and creativity can be experienced by the forensic patient as tormenting, provoking a sense of threat, activating primitive defences, destructiveness or both.

The forensic patient's relationship with the environment and the objects within it is one of exploitation and boundary violation, both as victim and as perpetrator. One of the first objectives of the dramatherapist therefore, and no different from other psychotherapists, is to provide conditions supportive to the emergence of a potential space within which the primitive defences and destructiveness can be contained, explored and reflected upon with the patient. Pedder (1977), making another link between psychotherapy and drama, tells us that: '...providing the space needed for psychotherapy, play or theatre has to be the responsibility of a trustworthy figure' (p.219).

The therapist in a forensic setting is unlikely to be viewed by the patient as a trustworthy figure, but perhaps something of this quality can develop by the therapist offering himself as: '...the guardian of a potential space in which meaning may arise' (Wright 1976, p.107).

I am here reminded also of Winnicott's statement: 'Psychotherapy has to do with two people playing together.' When a patient is not at all ready to play, the work of the therapist is: '...directed towards bringing the patient from a state of not being able to play into a state of being able to play' (1971, p.38).

With regard to two psychotherapists playing together, I note Duhl's (1999) thoughts that: 'Interaction between people includes not only words but also gestures, voice tones, body movements, pace, energy exchanges, and all the private meanings given these behaviours by each member involved' (p.80). In dramatherapy, the body as signifier moving in relation to a history of experience is an integral theme. As Jones (1996) states: 'For most forms of theatre and drama, in all cultures, the body is the main means of communication' (p.150).

CLINICAL EXAMPLE

I will now expand on these themes by turning to clinical material. I have in mind a male patient (P)[1] who was in treatment with me in once-weekly individual dramatherapy for six years; he was in his late thirties when our work began. P was an extremely damaged man, whose physical and sexual boundaries were, in childhood, repeatedly violated by adults and, when an adult himself, he felt the compulsion to repeat similar scenes in the role of perpetrator. In sessions P seemed able to inhabit the dramatherapy space only by showing me his need to keep moving. He roamed around the edges of the room and through the middle of the room, looking searchingly, suspiciously, covering as much of the floor space as was possible for him to do.

Along with P's roaming movement around and through the space came his verbal rants, targeted invariably at representations of authority. Intermittently he would seat himself on the chair provided, before standing again, unable to contain his impulse to move and unable to contain his use of the sessions as a place for discharging his rage. P's roaming and ranting seemed to effectuate each other, unable to neither rant without roaming nor roam without ranting. The rage was such that P could not include the concept of *other* and therefore could not enter into a therapeutic dialogue with me.

P had previously shown little sign of meaningful engagement with psychological therapies and his clinical team found him extremely difficult to communicate with. It had seemed impossible for P to work within the boundaries of verbal psychotherapy; equally, any invitation from me to facilitate an engagement to work within specific dramatherapy structures was experienced as an imposition. Any verbalised observation or interpretation from me was experienced as intrusive. P seemed able only to reject, needing to test the boundaries of my own capacity to be with him, and there were occasions when I certainly did struggle to be with him as his intense verbal onslaughts in the most turbulent sessions at times invoked a feeling of mental paralysis in me. This was an example of Bion's (1967) description of attacks on linking and thinking in action.

In trying to work out simply how to be with P, I improvised my response and began to accompany him in his movements, at the same time listening to and witnessing him giving physical form to his internal, unboundaried, conflict drama. I agree with Johnson (1991), who sees dramatherapy as a kind of psychoanalytic free association in action. I relate to what happened in the dramatherapy space as a piece of improvisational movement theatre, which brings to mind the theatre director Peter Brook's statement: 'I take an empty

---

1   I shall refer to the patient as P, whose clinical material has been disguised in order to respect confidentiality and protect anonymity.

space and call it a bare stage. A man walks across this empty space whilst someone else is watching him, and this is all that is needed for an act of theatre to be engaged' (1968, p.11). This kind of movement improvisation was what P and I engaged in, more or less, for practically the first three of the six years that I saw him. Incredibly in my experience with forensic patients, he never missed a session, neither did he give any indication of wanting to discontinue the therapy.

As I accompanied P's roaming movements around and through the therapeutic space he would stroke the walls with a shoulder, stopping at a window momentarily to look out of it, before roaming toward the window on the other side of the room; stopping for another moment to look inside a cupboard with a variety of objects such as masks and miniature figures but showing little curiosity in them. His pace was variable but it was more often a meandering pace with momentary bursts of quickness when he got particularly aroused. His body, though, was always tight and tense. Session after session I continued my roaming movement accompaniment: following his movement; sometimes matching his pace and quality; at other times I would counter him; I sometimes walked alongside him, or else moved away from him, creating space between us. At other times I would be still for a while, or lean against the wall. What came to mind for me was that it was as if a choreographic structure was being created by our two bodies in space. My movements were deliberately understated. My focus was on developing a physical eye, a physical intelligence, constantly placing my body in relation to P's body. Similar to a dance-movement improvisation of leader–follower, I allowed P to be the leader without him knowing that he was leading and I was therefore effectively following him. One can compare this to the process of a talking psychotherapy session with the psychotherapist following the journey of the patient, going where the patient takes the psychotherapist. The principle in this of course is that it is the follower who holds the boundaries. When I countered P's movement I was effectively making a movement proposal, which I see as a kind of interpretation, and like the analyst who waits to see what the patient will do with the interpretation, I waited to see what P did with each movement proposal. What he did was to move unremittingly through the therapeutic space but without awareness or feeling for it, concerned only in maintaining some sense of control over the space and to make the objects in it see, feel and sense his internal experience of chaotic unboundariedness. Over many months of sessions however, P slowly, and I need to emphasise slowly, started to respond physically, with his ranting diminishing concordantly. An example of this was that he began to move with me or towards me, accompanying some of my movement quality, joining me when I stood by the window or sat on the table. Stillness began to enter the therapeutic space and our physical relatedness became more *conversational.*

Discussion

I think that by moving in relation to P, I was extending the means whereby he and I could have a conversation. In sitting in the chair he could not speak directly from his experience, he could not have a conventional therapeutic conversation. By being *with* P I was trying to respond to him whereby he made a move and I responded. This, I think, helped to build a structure that could become a safe and contained enough holding environment. In other words the space became a different kind of relational field for him to be in, and what he was able to do eventually was to let something be seen and be more able to speak from something within him. One might call this embodied speech.

P's increasing experience was of the space being somewhat more trustworthy, and the dramatherapist being somewhat more trustworthy to be with, and he slowly became sufficiently minded about his own body to actually speak of his experience.

I am suggesting that it is the very act of being able to move around with P in this kind of dance, involving a movement and response relationship, that helped create boundaries. There were the physical boundaries of the room that were given, and there were psychological and emotional boundaries created and discovered between P and I. In the quality of the use of boundaries one finds meaning in containment, leading to the creation/discovery of a potential space. It was in this potential space, this in-between world, that P was able to let both me and himself know what was going on. I suggest it had to be in that play space otherwise it could not have happened, and the play space was given both by the formal dimensions of the room and by the therapeutic relationship that developed; the relationship between the physical boundaries of the room and the boundaries that were developed through the process of our collaboration together. That was the container. The container was the process.

The value of using my own body in this way was that it cultivated an awareness of a physical counter-transference. Hall (1992) writes: 'In the region of impoverished repertoire one role gets played over and over again, the script stays the same the subject never changes' (p.85). When P was roaming around the room and his movements repeated over and over again he was somatising the stuckness in his mind, imprisoned by a victim–perpetrator dynamic that he could not escape from unless he had it witnessed.

By my moving in relation to P I allowed myself to be used[2] in such a way that I had the experience of going through the same moves. In responding physically he received something in return – a different experience was being encountered by him. His somatised stuckness was being witnessed and collaborated with. An experience of having a witness was of great significance for P given that his childhood abuse was not believed by the adults he tried to turn to, leaving him to face his abuse alone again and again. A boy stuck between his abusers and his rejecters. This was what he needed to have witnessed, and to ensure that I believed him he needed to make it as real and as concrete as possible: repeatedly he had physically to show me. In following his repetitive roaming, together with his ranting, I had an experience of what it might have been like to have felt utterly controlled. P was letting me know what it felt like, but he was also letting me know how desperate he was to escape. By the process of being witnessed and responded to in his own idiom, his habitual roaming movement began to be invested with meaning and started to take on an explicit boundary – a process that took three years before he was able to move towards using the room and the objects in it in a different way, for instance, in thinking with me about the areas of the room that represented danger and the areas that represented safety. This representational use of the room brought with it a necessary acknowledgement of demarcations and boundaries. The room itself, then, the actual space, began to be used as a potential space for potential play.

Before these shifts came about, P's main mode of communication was through projective identification. It was important therefore to maintain a dramatherapeutic attitude, and I link this directly to an analytic attitude. Schafer's (1983) interpretation of Freud's papers on technique (1911–1915–1958) puts emphasis on furthering an atmosphere of safety as the overriding aim of the analytic attitude, and for interpretation to take place in a free-floating, non-directive way, providing an empathic connection and allowing for a space to be created in which something can emerge between patient and analyst/therapist. My dramatherapeutic attitude towards following, mirroring, countering, hint-taking, proposal-making movements is equivalent, I suggest, to an analytic attitude.

Many times I felt the provocation from P towards despair and rage, dismissive and abusive. It was at times a struggle to hold on to my own attitude, and it is here that the clinical supervisory space was a fundamental element to thinking about working with boundary phenomena in a forensic setting. It was in this triangular space, working with the third other, that thinking occurred, contributing to the safe and creative maintenance of therapeutic boundaries.

---

2   I am referring to Winnicott's (1953) meaning of the use of an object.

P later began to take up my proposal to make use of the variety of objects from the cupboard in the dramatherapy room. An example of this was his use of masks to depict his family. He looked at the masks and commented on their expressions, naming the emotions behind the expressions. P chose a mask that he thought represented a version of himself and went on to choose a different mask for each member of his family. I invited P to create a family sculpt with the masks. He took his time, slowly, deliberating thoughtfully on what he needed to create to best express what he needed to show. He placed the masks as closely bunched together as possible on the floor. I commented on my observation that there was little or no space between each mask/family member. He simply nodded his head. P went on to talk further and over many sessions he narrated the story of his family experiences to me.

It was through the use of the object masks, which began to carry a special quality and a meaning, that P started to tell his story. The masks were not-me objects used to refer to something in his life and the use of them helped to delineate the relationships in his family and he could begin to think about the claustrophobia that he encountered there. This process again promoted the creation/discovery of boundaries. The not-me objects were another element in the process to help P create the space that he was desperate to find in his internal world, enhancing his state of engagement towards play.

P was eventually able to use the dramatherapy space to reflect on his role as perpetrator; anxious though he was about this, he could allow enough stillness in his body and mind to permit thinking space. Although P's treatment was far from completed, he was deemed safe enough to move to lesser security.

CONCLUSION

I would like to close with the following quote: 'A feeling for drama and movement is likely to enrich the analytic process' (Wainwright [2010] 2013). In working with forensic patients the themes and issues of boundary phenomena will, in one shape or another, be ever-present. I have tried to illustrate one of the ways in which these dynamics present themselves in the dramatherapy work space, emphasising the importance of the therapist allowing himself to learn how to simply *be* with the patient when faced with a patient who cannot or will not *fit* into certain therapeutic boundaries set by the therapist. A feeling for drama, for movement, or art or music might indeed extend the practice of the talking therapies and allow further possibilities of reaching the patient.

REFERENCES

Bion, W.R. (1967) *Second Thoughts*. London: Karnac Books.

Brook, P. (1968) *The Empty Space*. London: Penguin Books.

Duhl, B.S. (1999) 'A Personal View of Action: Bringing What's Inside Outside.' In D.J. Weiner (ed.) *Beyond Talk Therapy: Using Movement and Expressive Techniques in Clinical Practice*. Washington DC: American Psychological Association.

Dunn Grayer, E. (2005) 'The Story of Alex – An Improvisational Drama.' *Clinical Social Work Journal 33* (Spring), 1, 21–36.

Freud, S. (1958) 'Papers On Technique (1911–1915).' In J. Strachey (ed.) *Standard Edition of the Complete Psychological Works of Sigmund Freud, Vol. 12*. London: Hogarth Press and The Institute of Psycho-Analysis.

Hall, N. (1992) 'Changing the Subject: Behind the Scenes in Psychotherapy's Theatre.' *Sphinx 4: A Journal for Archetypal Psychology and the Arts 81*, 104.

Johnson, D.R. (1991) 'The theory and technique of transformations in drama therapy.' *The Arts in Psychotherapy 18*, 285–300.

Jones, P. (1996) *Drama As Therapy: Theatre As Living*. London: Routledge.

McDougall, J. (1986) *Theatres of the Mind: Illusion and Truth on the Psychoanalytic Stage*. London: Free Association Books.

Ogden, T.H. (1985) 'On Potential Space.' *International Journal of Psychoanalysis 66*, 129–141.

Pedder, J.R. (1977) 'The Role of Space and Location in Psychotherapy, Play and Theatre.' *International Review of Psycho-Analysis 4*, 215–223.

Schafer, R. (1983) *The Analytic Attitude*. New York: Basic Books.

Wainwright, R. [2010] (2013) 'Learning to Move: Imagination in the Living Body.' Lecture given to the C.G Jung Public Lecture Series, Bristol, UK. To be published in D. Mathers (ed.) *Alchemy and Psychotherapy*. London: Routledge.

Winnicott, D.W. (1953) 'Transitional Objects and Transitional Phenomena – A Study of the First Not-Me Possession.' *International Journal of Psychoanalysis 34*, 89–97.

Winnicott, D.W. (1971) *Playing and Reality*. Hove: Brunner-Routledge.

Wright, K.J. (1976) 'Metaphor and Symptom: A Study of Integration and its Failure.' *International Review of Psycho-Analysis 3*, 97–109.

Chapter 7

DISCOVERING HARMONY: MUSIC THERAPY IN FORENSIC SETTINGS

Stella Compton Dickinson and Andy Benn

Overview

There are a range of recognized models in general music therapy practice. These have developed to meet the needs of specific client groups. The purpose of this chapter is to focus on boundary phenomena in the practice of forensic music therapy for patients receiving treatment in secure hospital settings. The authors will discuss boundary issues under several themes. Firstly, considering music therapy delivery within the context of the forensic setting, then with reference to clinical vignettes drawn from composite clinical material, looking at the inherent risks of treating patients who have committed violent offences. The chapter continues by exploring various issues of confidentiality, observation and time, followed by an explanation of how the intra-psychic world of the forensic patient may become apparent through jointly-created musical improvisation. The authors then explore some of the issues related to clinical supervision and to the musical recording of clinical material for this high-risk patient group, finally drawing the chapter to a close with a conclusion.

INTRODUCTION

Boundary crossings may occur in music therapy practice through the diverse therapeutic uses of music. Music per se is often viewed as recreational, either for private listening or within treatment as an expensive and limited resource which is not available to all. Music therapists, however, are frequently involved in wider projects, such as access to music outreach programmes. They are also often the central figure in bringing closed hospital communities together to create a musical performance.

Since the state registration of allied healthcare professionals was introduced in the United Kingdom in 1997, a clearer boundary has gradually become defined between recreational, psychological and educational use of music in health care. In the United Kingdom National Health Service (NHS), music therapists are qualified to postgraduate and masters levels. For employment in the NHS, registration with the Health Professions Council (HPC) is now mandatory. This ensures that standards of practice are upheld through continued professional development, through which music therapists are sufficiently skilled to deliver robust, psychologically based treatment in which improvised music or song writing is a central component.

The findings of the systematic review by Gold *et al.* (2005) were that music therapy is usually not tailored to specific diagnoses. Furthermore, therapy motivation in particular should be considered when prescribing and evaluating arts psychotherapies. These findings therefore support that mixed diagnoses groups are feasible. This in itself constitutes a boundary which has to be negotiated in the secure treatment setting because patients are usually categorized diagnostically. Wards are often designated for patients according to their psychiatric diagnoses. Separate services and ring-fenced funding exist for patients with severe and dangerous personality disorders.

The music therapist may therefore have to negotiate the crossing of administrative boundaries based on diagnosis, in order to create a mixed diagnoses group drawn from several wards, or otherwise accept the geographical limitations and develop on-ward groups. These can be less contained than when using an identified music therapy room and they are not common in high secure treatment. The ward-based group can pose additional risks of envious attacks from patients who are unable to engage. Staff may also be negatively affected by the sounds that can often be heard outside the identified therapy 'space'. Those on the outside of the group will not fully understand the overall content or meaning of the musical communication. They may also feel excluded by not knowing the related verbal content or emotional issues that are being explored within the music medium.

Music therapy can be perceived as an attractive and complementary addition to standard multi-disciplinary treatments. Without sufficient explanatory liaison work on the part of the music therapist it can, however, be misperceived by other clinicians in the team. This has the potential to lead to further boundary transgressions and inappropriate referrals. An example of one of the most challenging reasons for referral received was simply given as 'multiple murders'. In fact the patient so referred benefited very well, having found a medium in which he could express his emotions and find a more authentic inner voice through his musical self-expression. The nature of the referral, though, indicates that the clinical team had exhausted the range of interventions available to the patient who was regarded as 'long-term treatment-resistant'. They were prepared to give anything a try to create inner change and this required careful risk assessment to ensure the safety of both the therapist and the patient.

RISK

For their own safety, staff in secure treatment settings must comply with hospital policies and procedures. Within a closed living environment these procedures, along with an intensive multi-disciplinary approach in which patients receive a range of concurrent treatments, can present a challenge in delivering effective therapy. Consideration has to be given to context-specific models through which the helpful ingredients of music therapy can remain available to the patient, despite the constraints of the setting.

Risk procedures exist to ensure the safety of staff and patients, the latter of whom have committed serious offences. This can sometimes be difficult to keep in mind when actively engaged in developing a therapeutic rapport through subjective interactive music-making. The risks of harm to both staff and patient are of the highest concern for multi-disciplinary teams. All staff receive mandatory security training as part of their induction, so this should occur prior to starting any clinical work.

One of the purposes of secure hospital risk management procedures is to have a controlling, yet containing, effect. Within the walls of the usually more remote settings of the high secure hospitals in the UK, the effect is of a surprisingly calm, quiet and safe environment. Balancing the necessary security procedures with safe and compassionate treatment is a constant organizational concern.

For these vulnerable yet volatile patients, if risk procedures are imposed too rigorously, for example through excessively anxious staff responses, the patient may feel overly controlled and restricted, rather than just safe.

If patients become distressed, staff have to manage the potential risk of dangerous and impulsive behaviour. Lack of control over impulsivity is a key factor which in many cases led to the offence committed by a person suffering from a serious and enduring mental disorder. Risk procedures therefore place a necessary boundary on how therapy can be delivered and how organizational security procedures are applied in the delivery of therapy.

For example, in order to physically get to the therapy room, patients receive 'pat down' searches from a member of staff who is of the same sex. This occurs before they are escorted from their ward to the music therapy room, and then again prior to returning and re-entering their ward. Therefore, in the music therapy room, to ensure that no items have been concealed, an inventory of musical equipment will be taken at the start and end of therapy sessions. The risk is that music therapy instruments could be perceived as 'weapons', or made into weapons. However, clinical experience suggests that the therapeutic containment provided by an identified therapy room may mitigate the risk of patients acting in this way.

When in the music therapy room, physical contact with patients is inevitably limited. There is a risk that touch may create sexual arousal and a desire for intimacy. This is a complex issue that requires thought and discussion. The patient who has been through the criminal justice system may already perceive himself as stigmatized and to be untouchable. The therapist's stance naturally should not constitute a reinforcement of feelings of exclusion and shame, neither should it be over-compensatory and comforting, which could lead to seductive fantasies and a counter-therapeutic, very dangerous situation. The therapist must therefore decide on an appropriate and consistent stance regarding how to greet their patients and how to say goodbye at the end of sessions.

Commonly, patients who have offended oscillate between victim and offender states of being. Multiple issues, including feelings of shame, can make it difficult for the patient to look at the darker side of his personality and therefore to engage in work on the index offence. Offence-related work is only undertaken when the multi-disciplinary team consider that the patient is at the right stage in his overall treatment pathway to address these issues. The risk is that current circumstances or therapeutic material raised to consciousness may resonate with, and trigger a reactivation of, the thoughts, feelings and behaviours that constitute the patient's offender state of being. This increases the risk of re-offending and is counter-therapeutic if the patient engages in offence-paralleling behaviours within the hospital setting.

In music therapy there is greater opportunity for physical movement and exploration within the therapy room, than is available in a purely talking therapy. Offence-related behaviours may therefore surface and can be observed in the symbolic use of instruments. For example continuous, loud playing on the drum kit can preclude any hope of a musical dialogue and thereby potentially overwhelm the therapist. Pointing or stabbing actions with the beaters can feel accusatory and attacking. This behaviour can be a form of symbolic offence re-enactment, which may be underpinned by violent fantasies. Therefore further consideration is required regarding the patient's motivation and how to develop his self-awareness.

These potentially provocative actions, whilst providing a cathartic effect for the patient, can usually be named in a non-judgemental manner. The purpose of subtly highlighting to the patient the impact of his behaviour on the therapist is to ascertain his level of insight; and by so doing to consider whether he really wants to annihilate his therapist with attacking sounds, or alternatively whether his musical expression may help him to develop his self-awareness regarding the impact of his behaviour on others. This gradual process has the potential to lead towards new and healthy feelings of remorse, particularly if a positive therapeutic alliance has already been established with the patient. He may then be dismayed that his behaviour could be perceived as damaging to his therapist. In this way, his pushing of the boundaries can be safely resolved as he develops greater self-awareness. Risk and observation procedures are therefore necessary in forensic work but in themselves constitute an additional boundary which is far more rigid than is the norm in community-based treatment.

Once the risks reduce to a point where high secure care is no longer appropriate, the care pathway out of high security hospitals for most patients is via a medium secure unit. One of the purposes of the patient's move from high to medium secure treatment is to assess and observe how he may respond to more flexible boundaries, including through greater access to the community and to the general public. This involves carefully calculated risk management in medium secure treatment as access to the community begins and thereby more freedom is experienced.

CONFIDENTIALITY, OBSERVATION AND TIME

In conditions of lesser security, therapists are usually required to escort their patients from the ward to the therapy room. This presents challenges in terms of how to maintain the confidential boundaries of the session and at what point the session begins. Therefore the time boundary requires reinforcement regarding when the process has actually started, along with consideration of what may feel mutually safe to talk about outside the confidential space provided by the therapy room. In high secure treatment settings the therapist must be prepared to accommodate the observation of sessions by nursing escort staff. There are positive and potentially negative implications to consider.

The therapist's ability to reflect, negotiate with and guide staff is required in order to hold the confidentiality of the space. Whilst working as part of a multi-disciplinary team, the therapist is responsible for holding the space and containing and acknowledging the emotions that may be elicited in the patient through close observation. Staff observation for the safety of all concerned may in fact put a patient who has suffered prior abuse in a supposedly private room at greater ease; alternatively, if mishandled, observation may feel uncomfortably voyeuristic.

Some hospitals have designated patient escort nursing staff (who often pride themselves on supporting the patient to attend and engage in their sessions). Music therapists can build up their professional relationships with these members of staff, who in turn are afforded an opportunity to learn more about the therapeutic approach. A sound relationship between the music therapist and escorting nursing staff, which has to build up over time, enables the music therapist to contain the therapeutic relationship within the confines of the therapy room.

One positive aspect of observed sessions is that the music therapist is included as a member of the multi-disciplinary team. Isolation of the music therapist from the clinical team can become a boundary distortion if a collusion develops through which the therapist becomes split off from the rest of the team and targeted by a predatory patient. In such a situation the therapist becomes the prey to the predator. This violation of boundaries will fatally rupture the therapeutic relationship. Therefore, for the safety of all concerned, there must be an agreement at the start of treatment regarding what is shared with the multi-disciplinary team. The patient must be aware that continuous multi-disciplinary notes are kept, through which clinicians can access each other's entries. This is of course an entirely different boundary in which clinical information is shared within the team, which is quite unlike the tighter boundaries of confidentiality in the context of private clinical practice.

Any perceived risks of dangerous behaviour as observed in therapy sessions are discussed with attendant staff afterwards and in confidence. It is all too easy for misunderstandings to occur between what an external observer sees but cannot hear and the therapist's capacity to contain and process therapy material. Communication is vital yet a sensitive issue, after sessions, the purpose of which is to clarify and discuss different perceptions, yet without breaking the developing therapeutic alliance.

Observational procedures may result in greater resistance in the patient to developing a therapeutic alliance. However, empirical clinical evidence suggests that observation can also support a steadier pace through which the patient is able to access repressed psychological material and make relevant disclosures without the reactivation of trauma. A developmental psychodynamic approach can provide a gentle pace over years, by which patients can have a sense of continuity whilst other time-limited, specific offence-related treatments are started and completed. This is demonstrated in a long-term case by Compton Dickinson and Souflas (2011).

When the clinical and the managerial (fund-holding) teams under the leadership of the responsible clinician can support long-term music therapy, this can enable the patient to access deeper psychological material, and to safely work through negative transferences, as demonstrated by Glyn (2003), thereby hopefully developing more effective relating strategies in the present. An example of a re-enactment of offence-related behavior is given by Sleight in her experiences as co-therapist in Compton Dickinson and Sleight (2012).

The patient may feel reassured if the music therapist works closely with his named nurse. These boundaries require careful consideration regarding what is brought to and held in therapy and how much nursing support is appropriate or available to support the patient to process therapy material between sessions. It can be helpful for the patient to witness a cohesive approach, with the therapist and nurse working together from their individual perspectives rather than employing divergent approaches between the interventions.

In high secure treatment, the therapy sessions for patients with dangerous and severe personality disorders are usually attended and observed by a member of nursing staff present in the therapy room for the duration of the session. Different members of staff may be allocated to observe the music therapy sessions from week to week. This depends on the pre-planned nursing rotas and can make continuity and confidentiality in therapy much more difficult. In these circumstances the music therapist is required to think flexibly and assess the appropriate amount of involvement in therapy sessions from members of the nursing team. An important consideration is the degree of comfort and spontaneity with the musical medium that individual staff members in attendance may express. Too much nursing staff engagement can impair rather than encourage the patient to engage and thus the therapeutic boundary is transgressed. Alternatively if the nurse feels very self-conscious this may detrimentally affect the dynamics in the room. The therapist has to consider how best to put the nurse at ease and enable them to do their job in promoting a safe and facilitating environment.

To consider an effective patient–therapist match, based on the patient's unique history, personality and psychopathology, requires consideration in supervision alongside consideration of the level of experience of the music therapist. Their clinical placement experience rarely incorporates high secure settings, due to the inherent risks and long induction process prior to direct patient contact. Therefore the therapist's ability to hold the therapeutic boundaries with such extremely perverse and severely damaged individuals is relatively untried until they are employed in post.

Time-limited treatments are frequently intensive in content. The pressure to move patients through their treatment pathways, due to the very high cost of high secure treatment, often necessitates a time limit and the achievement of agreed therapy objectives; therefore an identifiable outcome is expected. In lower secure settings, after months during which formal processes are completed, patients may leave the unit with little notice or preparation for closure.

The time limits in forensic treatment are therefore frequently prescriptive rather than tailored to the pace of each patient's development. The latter may occur more commonly in private practice. Working to a prescribed time limit requires a careful balancing act and collaboration with the patient and team, to agree what might be achievable within each patient's capacity over the given period of time. Without this consideration, there is a risk that deep and potentially traumatic material is accessed too soon, prior to the development of sufficient ego strength.

THE INTRA-PSYCHIC WORLD OF THE PATIENT

This section will explore how the patient's internal states of confusion and chaos may be externalized through the process of musical improvisation in a clinical setting, thereby creating the potential for boundary transgressions and readjustments.

Central to forensic psychotherapy is the nature of the index offence. Music therapy has the potential to enhance specific offence-focused psychology programmes. These are frequently based in cognitive behavioural, cognitive analytic or dialectical behavioural models. Consideration of the offence, whilst frequently not named in sessions, remains central in the music therapist's thinking when working towards facilitating the patient's ability to safely access and recognize previously unconscious responses.

Whilst music therapy does not frequently constitute explicit offence-related work, the implicit and frequently intimate nature of making music has the potential to expand the patient's emotional range of expression and engagement in relation to his offence. The patient's inner states can often be heard within his jointly created music, during which he may access and express his emotions in response to the therapist in a dialogical exchange. He is then no longer alone with these difficult or previously unacceptable feelings. These emotions can then be named, thereby increasing self-awareness. The patient may subsequently be able to re-avow previously dissociated experiences to his consciousness. The recognition and reintegration of these previously split-off and disavowed self-states can occur when both memory and emotion are actively engaged (Compton Dickinson 2006). Thus, boundaries are re-ordered in aiming for a more integrated development of the self.

As treatment progresses, patients may experience archaic feelings of anxiety, the symptoms of which can impair their global functioning. The ability to explore may mean that the patient's mental health appears to deteriorate before getting better. However, this may amount to increased insight into anxious behaviours and internal change, rather than deterioration. There is always the risk that this situation may be viewed by the team as a potentially detrimental one. It may be difficult for nursing staff to understand these changes and also to manage apparently deteriorated mental health and concomitant increased risk-behaviours on a ward. The music therapist requires considerable robustness and refined interpersonal skills to contain team anxieties as well as those of the patient. The music therapy treatment emphasis is often aimed towards the patient's ability to develop a wider range of responses that are creatively and aesthetically pleasing, through which he may increase his insight into his oppositional, destructive behaviours. The latter may otherwise be acted out in violent and callous use of the instruments as objects, rather than perceiving them as vibrant, alive means of self-expression. The music therapist might decide to respond by supporting the patient's identification with particular instruments which can become like 'friends' to the patient. One patient made 'friends' with the large Tam Tam Gong. She gave it a name, as this rotund instrument brought up reminders of a relative who had suffered an accident and then, having been thin, became very fat. Through this association with accidents and old connections, links were made and parallel processes to the patient's own life explored.

Anger and frustration can be appropriately and safely expressed through supported musical improvisation. For example, the therapist may decide to play intentionally discordant music to mirror the disturbed feelings of the patient's inner world as perceived through the counter-transference. This can then be gradually mediated through skilful improvisational techniques whereby the patient's mood becomes more smoothly moderated to a calmer state which feels more acceptable to both patient and therapist. Yet throughout the improvisation, the patient should be able to retain a sense of shared ownership of the musical creation.

If a patient's offence involved the indecent assault of a woman he may respond to a female music therapist either through fear of intimacy, for example by creating greater distance, as in one case, by intentionally playing out of tune; or in subversive and predatory ways through which he may attempt to subtly seduce the therapist by eliciting pity and presenting himself as the helpless, abused child victim. Such ingrained behaviours are a form of symbolic offence re-enactment in which grooming was learnt by the patient at an early age, through the process of identification with his abuser. To continue to repeat such behaviour is counter-therapeutic and can be differentiated from positively negotiated creative expression through the negative emotions which can be felt as subtly present in the therapy room. Destructive, mocking, or rejecting reciprocal roles (Ryle and Kerr 2002) may be enacted in particular within group improvisation. These often represent negative reciprocations of the patient's own past experience with peers, in which he may have been mocked or humiliated: as demonstrated in Compton Dickinson and Sleight (2011).

In cognitive analytic terminology (Ryle and Kerr 2002), these enactments and relating patterns are understood as reciprocal roles, the recognition of which is required to avoid the perpetuation of an unhealthy collusion. Collusion is risky but it may occur in musical improvisation if a war like dialogue strays from containment to that of an all-out musical battle between individuals fighting for the upper hand, frequently feeling controlled or seeking to take control. This may have a useful therapeutic impact if the therapist understands what is happening and the collusion can be recognized, shared and understood by both therapist and patient and therefore resolved. If this does not occur, the boundary into the patient's inner world has been crossed without returning safety to a reality-orientated state. The potential and risks involved in the offence-related qualities of non-verbal communications, as enacted in improvised music, as well as the verbal communications, should be unravelled in supervision.

A three-way inter-disciplinary approach is possible when the music therapist's integration with the nursing team is strong and cohesive. There are pros and cons in considering whether one can work from an object relations perspective and involve the staff member as a positive role model. Consistent nurse and therapist relationships with the patient can provide a sense of continuity for a mentally disturbed patient who may have never experienced any positive role modelling (Compton Dickinson 2012; Adlam and Odell-Miller 2012). If this is achieved, early dysfunctional parenting experiences can be reworked as the patient becomes a witness to staff collaboration and positive role modelling, thereby creating a corrective therapeutic experience for the patient.

The choice of treatment approach is influenced by the severity of the index offence and the duration of the therapy. For example, over time dangerous oedipal fantasies may surface through transference-related issues. The index offence is considered in the context of transference-based therapy. The majority of forensic patients have come from disturbed family backgrounds where they have experienced domestic violence. For example, if the patient witnessed a murder as a child, or committed matricide, the same thoughts, fears and responses could be reactivated through a positive maternal transference in music therapy. This area is fraught with complex issues that require multi-disciplinary discussion. If the symbolic nature of the transference is lost with a psychotic patient, perhaps within what may feel like comforting and attuned musical improvisation, then the boundary between who the therapist really is and what the patient is yearning or grieving for becomes blurred, thereby putting the therapist at risk of a psychotic transference pervaded by concrete thinking.

Glyn (2009) warns against the risks of triangulation through which dangerous oedipal fantasies may result if the therapist is misperceived by the patient to be collaborating intimately with another staff member. The result may be a lack of trust in the confidentiality of the session, or primitive feelings of envy may be activated in the patient. This creates a highly toxic situation in which the patient may want what the other has got at any cost, even to a point of seeking to destroy the object of envy.

CLINICAL SUPERVISION AND RECORDING

Clinical supervision is the essential objective requirement in gaining an external qualitative viewpoint of processes within the music therapy process. The therapist is unable to help the patient to recognize the impact of his behaviours on others without firstly recognizing and gaining understanding for herself of the meaning of these communications, and the processes and enactments that are occurring in the therapy room. The qualitative and subjective nature of making music can be difficult or deceptive to evaluate in the therapy sessions and some distance is gained on the process by reflecting more safely in supervision (Odell-Miller and Richards 2009).

The therapist is generally more inclined to see the child/victim self-state of the patient, because the nature of the index offence can make it difficult to hold in mind the perversity and horror of the patient's offence. Without a balanced objective view through supervision there can also be a risk of an erotic transference developing, particularly with young and beautiful therapists, in which unconscious and conscious seductive processes could develop to undermine the therapeutic outcome as well as putting the therapist at risk.

An important safeguard for the therapist rests in developing skills to work with the counter-transference, through which one's own bodily and intuitive feelings inform the therapist of the patient's internal state. Projective identification remains a risk by which the therapist may act on behalf of the patient's own projected thoughts. Frequently this may not become apparent until supervision or after considerable reflective work in peer group supervision.

As a standard consent procedure, music therapy improvisations are usually recorded. This enables objective assessment by both therapist and patient as well as the development of the therapist's skills and the therapeutic process. A patient-centred approach can be maintained by listening to the recordings; however, recording is not always possible, depending on the mental state of the patient, particularly if a patient has psychotic delusions. This issue can be navigated through a careful assessment process whereby early sessions may not be recorded until a therapeutic alliance and trust have been established. Recording may then start when a treatment phase is agreed and a rapport has developed. The therapist has therefore to negotiate with the multi-disciplinary team at what point a patient has sufficient mental stability to start therapy.

The advantage of recording the improvisations only, rather than verbal input also, enables both patient and therapist to reflect together on their jointly created music. This can help to develop rapport. The fact that the music is jointly created makes music therapy unique in that the therapist is more than a witness to the process – they are actively involved in a subjective process, which enables the therapist to enter the patient's inner world, to support the patient to express himself. Ultimately the musical improvisation needs to return to a safe place. Likewise the recording must be kept in a safe place. There is the potential of misuse of the recording if either patient or therapist remove it from the premises, so boundaries are set regarding consent to record and not to make profit or commercial gain from the use of recorded therapeutic material.

The different states of being in patients who have offended can usefully be heard in the qualitative aspects of musical improvisations. Self-states are common in patients who have offended and who have personality disorder. These are best described by Pollock et al. (2001). The self-states model was conceptualized by Ryle (1997). He described borderline personality states of being as often partially dissociated, though they may be fully dissociated and disconnected from each other, particularly in the case of a person who has committed a violent offence, and therefore indicative of dissociative identity disorder (ICD-10 F44.8, World Health Organization, 1992). For example, in narcissistic personality disorder the individual may fluctuate suddenly and dangerously from a self-state in which he may feel superior, ruthless and contemptuous to feeling utterly 'punctured', inferior and contemptible. This may be played out musically, for example, by a total disregard of the therapist's attempt to connect, if the patient is in a callous and darkly dangerous 'offender' state; alternatively the patient may expresses his neglected, lost child state, represented by sorrowful desperate cries, often choosing to play the whistle or recorder. Fear may be expressed in high, teetering piano playing, with the quality of the music describing an internal state which may be both indecisive and frightened. In these ways powerful emotions are accessed which may give a unique insight into the patient's mental state, even to a point of suicidal ideation, which without the use of music may have been missed. Viewed in this way, the qualitative, musical aspects of supervision can be beneficial for both patient and supervisee in holding the boundaries.

The therapist may have to address their own narcissistic desire to fix a patient and their own issues of loss which may be touched through those of her patient. Another purpose of supervision is to create balance, thereby restoring internal harmony through which the therapist can differentiate patient and personal material which may have been activated, and remain separate and objective from the patient. In this way the therapist can hold her boundaries and retain the focus on the patient's material, without the frequently profound levels of patient need becoming overwhelming or pervading her work-lifestyle balance.

CONCLUSION

Music therapy practice varies between high, medium and low secure hospital settings. There is as yet little rigorous outcome research on music therapy in forensic settings. The current drive is towards acceptable, evidence-based, context-specific models of treatment which can be incorporated successfully into the overall multi-disciplinary treatment pathways.

Observation procedures pose a challenge for music therapists in how to effectively engage patients who are frequently treatment-resistant. Therapeutic techniques may have to be modified to meet organizational expectations and the multi-disciplinary overall task.

Patients in secure treatment have a right to expect evidence-based treatments (Duggan *et al.* 2007). Assessment and treatment is directed towards rehabilitation and recovery. Qualitative evidence of psychological change for the better is expected in the NHS system, in order to validate the expense. Through a systematic approach, ideally following medical research council (MRC) guidance for the development of complex interventions, the active ingredients of music therapy can be identified, and qualitatively and quantitatively tested. The future of forensic music therapy lies in developing this evidence base and a broad range of clinically effective models.

REFERENCES

Antisocial Personality Disorder. The NICE Guidelines of Treatment, Management and Prevention (2009) National Clinical Practice Guideline Number 77, National Collaborating Centre for Mental Health Commissioned by the National Institute for Clincal Excellence. London: The British Psychological Society and The Royal College of Psychiatrists.

Compton Dickinson, S. (2006) 'Beyond Body, Beyond Words: Cognitive analytic music therapy in forensic psychiatry – New approaches in the treatment of personality disordered offenders.' *Music Therapy Today 11*, 4, 839–875. Available at http://musictherapyworld.net, accessed on 23 February 2012.

Compton Dickinson, S.J. & Sleight, V. (2012) 'Group Cognitive Analytic Music Therapy (G-CAMT): A developmental pilot group for men who have killed or committed grievous bodily harm'. In J. Adam, S.J. Compton Dickinson and H. Odell-Miller (eds) *Forensic Music Therapy*. London: Jessica Kingsley Publishers.

Compton Dickinson, S.J. and Souflas, P. (2011) 'Rapping Round the System: A Young Black Man's Journey through a High Secure Hospital'. In S. Hadley and G. Yancy ((eds) *Therapeutic Uses of Rap and Hip Hop*'. New York: Routledge.

Compton Dickinson, S.J., Adlam, J. and Odell-Miller, H. (2012) 'A case of work, rest and play: music therapy in early onset psychosis.' In *Forensic Music Therapy*. London: Jessica Kingsley Publishers.

Duggan, C., Adams, C., McCarthy, L., Fenton, M. *et al.* (2007) 'A Systematic Review of the Effectiveness of Pharmacological and Psychological Treatments for those with Personality Disorder.' Nottinghamshire Healthcare NHS Trust Institute of Mental Health.

Glyn, J. (2003) 'New York Mining Disaster.' *British Journal of Music Therapy 17*, 2, 97.

Glynn, J. (2009) 'Two's company, three's a crowd. Hatred of triangulation in music therapy in the forensic setting.' In H. Odell-Miller and E. Richards (eds) *Supervision of Music Therapy*. London: Routledge.

Gold, C., Heldal, T.O., Dahle, T. and Wigram, T. (2005) 'Music therapy for schizophrenia-like illnesses.' *The Cochrane Database Systemic Reviews 2005*, Issue 2. Art. No. CN004025.pub2. DOI: 10.1002/14651858.cd004025.pub2.

Odell-Miller, H. and Richards, E. (eds) (2009) *Supervision of Music Therapy*. London: Routledge.

Pollock, P.H., Broadbent, M., Clarke, S., Dorrian, A. and Ryle, A. (2001) 'Assessment. The Personality Structure Questionnaire (PSQ): A Measure of the Multiple Self States Model of Identity Disturbance in Cognitive Analytic Therapy.' *Clinical Psychology and Psychotherapy 6*, 59–72.

Ryle, A. (1997) *Cognitive Analytic Therapy and Borderline Personality Disorder*. Chichester: John Wiley & Sons.

Ryle, A. and Kerr, I. (2002) *Introducing Cognitive Analytic Therapy*. Chichester: John Wiley & Sons.

World Health Organization (1992) *International Statistical Classification of Diseases and Related Health Problems* (ICD-10). Geneva: WHO.

APPENDIX

The Oxford Dictionary definition of a boundary is a 'line which marks the limits of an area; a dividing line'. Also included is the suggestion that a boundary can be the 'limit of something abstract, especially a subject or sphere of activity'. The latter suggests both internal, unspoken as well as external, concrete concepts. As such, it may be a good point from which to begin to explore the professional and therapeutic boundaries when delivering music therapy in a forensic treatment setting.

Curiously, the origin of the word boundary, which goes back to the seventeenth century, is a variant of 'bounder', the meaning of which suggests behaviour which goes beyond that which is acceptable. This could also be applied to patients in a high secure hospital, all of whom have committed an offence going beyond the boundaries of acceptable social norms. They are admitted to a secure hospital through the criminal justice system following their conviction, at which point massive external boundaries are in place to ensure that they cannot escape.

Chapter 8

WORKING WITH FAMILIES IN FORENSIC SETTINGS: A SYSTEMIC PERSPECTIVE ON BOUNDARIES

Jo Bownas

Overview

In this chapter I will introduce aspects of working with boundaries in family therapy in a medium secure inpatient setting. The chapter will be built around a clinical vignette. To protect confidentiality, the family described is not a 'real' family but a composite of families the family therapy team have worked with, representing themes and actual events we have encountered in our work. I will begin by introducing the vignette and then refer to some relevant theory, relating it to the family presented in the vignette. Finally I will describe how the work with the family unfolded. Within the constraints of a short chapter, therapeutic time is collapsed and the result does not do justice to the messiness of therapy: the frustrations, false starts and failures of which we certainly have our share. Nor does it acknowledge adequately the developments that, in our setting, might be taking place simultaneously in other areas of the patient's treatment and the effect these developments may have on the progress of family therapy. Nevertheless, I hope the chapter will give the reader a glimpse at some of the theories, practices and intentions of family therapy approaches to working with boundaries in a forensic setting.

CASE VIGNETTE: THE KAPOOR FAMILY

Pallab Kapoor is a thirty-year-old man of Indian heritage. Born in London, he grew up with his three sisters and his parents, who migrated to Britain after their marriage. His father has his own business and his mother works part time in catering. His sisters are all now married and living nearby. Pallab achieved average results in GCSEs but quickly dropped out of A level college and had a series of short-term jobs. He began drinking alcohol and using cannabis in his mid-teens and later experimented with other drugs. He continued living with his parents. At the age of 27, Pallab attacked a neighbour, leaving him seriously injured. He was found to be experiencing acute psychotic symptoms with delusional beliefs about the neighbour. After a period in prison he was transferred to hospital, where he remained after sentencing, on a Hospital Order with Restrictions (S37/41). Pallab has made a good recovery from his psychotic symptoms but the multi-disciplinary team (MDT) looking after him is concerned about his lack of motivation for his therapeutic programme and his tendency to minimise the seriousness of his offence and his illness.

In talking about his life Pallab describes a strict upbringing in which he was expected to concentrate on his studies to the exclusion of play and friendships. He was close to his mother but fearful of his father, who had high expectations and a quick temper. Pallab describes his parents as ignoring his later substance misuse, while pressuring him to get a good job and to marry. The MDT believe that Pallab's family may now be contributing to difficulties in his treatment through their 'over-involvement'. Mr and Mrs Kapoor visit their son every day. Mrs Kapoor does Pallab's washing for him and brings him food at every visit. The MDT fears that this is undermining their attempts to help Pallab develop more independence and the skills of self-care. From their contact with the family they also suspect that the family supports Pallab in minimising the seriousness of his offence and discourages him from involvement in parts of the therapeutic programme aimed at addressing substance misuse and offending behaviour. They ask the Family Work Team for help.

When we met with the MDT they identified their concern about a number of possible boundary issues:

- Lack of an appropriate boundary between Pallab and his mother may be fostering dependence and impeding Pallab's development.

- The boundary between Pallab and his father may maintain Mr Kapoor as the (harsh and demanding) authority in Pallab's life, limiting his autonomy and generating in Pallab an unexpressed and potentially dangerous resentment.

- Mr and Mrs Kapoor are experienced at violating the boundaries of the institution: they visit over-regularly and perform tasks (feeding and laundry) which are usually managed by the institution; and they seem to support their son in not engaging with important aspects of his treatment.

- Pallab's parents seem to have imposed over-rigid boundaries on him in childhood, limiting his social development, and later failed to impose appropriate boundaries around his behaviour in adolescence and early adulthood.

- Pallab's index offence represents a criminal breach of the boundaries of socially acceptable behaviour. The team is concerned that he and his family do not view this breach with sufficient seriousness.

How do we approach these issues in family therapy?

A LITTLE THEORY AND PRACTICE

Contexts and circles

Family therapy is founded on the idea that human relationships are a *context* for understanding individual experience and actions (Watzlawick, Beavin Bavelas and Jackson 1967). The MDT's referral above shows that they share that idea: they think that the worrying behaviours shown by Pallab may be influenced and explained by his relationship with his parents. The individual is influenced by the circumstances and relationships which form their context at a given point in time; and their responses in turn influence those circumstances and relationships, in a circular fashion. This *circularity* is another key systemic concept. It leads us not just to think about how Pallab's family may be a context for *his* actions and beliefs, but to consider how in turn his actions influence his *family*. And so, when we meet with Pallab and his family, our focus is on the *relationship* between people, rather than on individuals.

The idea of circularity points to another systemic concept: *punctuation*. Punctuation refers to the selection of a particular viewpoint from which to describe or explain interactions. So, punctuated from Pallab's point of view, the story of his early family relationships is of a lonely child, longing for friendship and play and emotionally distanced from his family by the demands of an authoritarian father. From the father's viewpoint the story may appear differently: he may describe working hard to give his children the best opportunities through a good education, intensifying his efforts as he sees the children being influenced by a culture which threatens to alienate them from their family. Thus, in systemic work, we are interested in *multiple perspectives*, rather than in a singular 'truth' (e.g. Jones 1993). We are interested in the richer picture that emerges from multiple perspectives and in how these different views might interact together. For instance it may be that the more demanding Pallab's father became, the more Pallab was drawn to life outside the family; and the more Pallab sought to be involved in extra-familial activities and relationships, the more restrictive the father became, reinforcing the family's boundaries. Similarly, if we punctuate the relationship between the family and the hospital from the point of view of the MDT, we see the family as breaching the boundaries of the institution. But from the viewpoint of the family it is likely that they see the institution as breaching *their* boundaries by removing their son and taking over their functions of care and moral guidance. Again a circular and escalating pattern may emerge: the institution seeks to reinforce its boundaries and the family responds by intensifying their efforts to retain their own boundary, keeping their son within it; the institution experiences this as further intrusion by the family, and responds by drawing a yet more restrictive boundary around the family's involvement.

Family boundaries

Minuchin (1974) proposed that family 'structure' – rules governing family organisation, patterns of interaction and hierarchies of power and authority – was an important context for the development of family members. For Minuchin, a significant element of family structure is the maintenance of appropriate boundaries between individual family members and between 'sub-systems' (e.g. parents may be thought of as one sub-system and children as another within the family system; there may be a father-and-son sub-system; or a teenagers sub-system). In this model, if boundaries are either too rigid or too diffuse they may become a context for problems to emerge; and the structural family therapist aims to help the family establish (or re-establish) boundaries that are clear but flexible enough to adapt to changing demands on the family and individual members. Other systemic approaches (including the Milan, Post-Milan and Social Constructionist approaches that have particularly influenced my own practice) have theorised family systems differently; but questions of belonging and separation, closeness and distance, and the operation of power and authority are recurring themes for all of us. We will see later how these themes emerged in our work with the Kapoor family.

Extending our understanding of boundaries

In its early stages of development the focus of family therapy was on the 'system' of the family, viewed as contained within its own boundaries and amenable to objective observation and expert intervention by the therapist. Significant developments in the field later extended the boundaries of the therapist's attention. Therapists began to realise that focusing on the family in isolation meant ignoring significant relationships (e.g. friends, colleagues, professional helpers) and significant contexts (e.g. the family's culture, ethnicity, economic circumstances). Boscolo *et al.* (1987) for instance, describe moving from thinking about the family system to considering the *significant system*, which they see as including all the people and institutions connected to the problem or to attempted solutions. So, we may think of Pallab's significant system as including not just his family but also the hospital and the relationships he has with professionals and other patients.

Including the therapist in the significant system

In a parallel development, second-order cybernetics (e.g. Boscolo *et al.* 1987) challenged the idea that the therapist could stand outside the system and led us to consider how the family is influenced by the presence of the therapist. The later influence of social constructionism (e.g. McNamee and Gergen 1992) took us further away from the idea of an individual or family as having a single stable identity and towards considering how those identities are constructed differently in interactions in a host of interweaving social contexts. As therapists, then, we think about how we can relate with the family in ways that invite them to be their preferred selves; how we can construct a relationship that has the potential to be *collaborative* and generative. Thus, for example, when we met with Pallab and his parents we encouraged talk about aspects of their life not marked by problems and pathology, such as Mr Kapoor's successful business, Mrs Kapoor's ability to combine work and caring for her grandchildren and Pallab's interest in the progress of his nieces and nephews. In this way we hoped to invite a *positioning* (Davies and Harre 1990) of the family as competent, moral and respected adults in our conversations.

On boundaries, blame and change

In keeping with Boscolo *et al.* (1987) we believe that it is harder to change under a negative connotation (when our actions and intentions are negatively judged). We are also influenced by Griffith and Elliot Griffith (1994) who note the potential silencing effect of hierarchies of power. In a forensic mental health setting opportunities for negative connotation abound. Pallab has breached boundaries of socially acceptable behaviour and the boundaries of the law, as well as being diagnosed with mental illness; and his family is likely to have become caught up in the potentially stigmatising search for explanation and attribution of blame. In this setting, hierarchies of power are also starkly visible, as the institution is charged with responsibility for restricting Pallab's liberty and imposing on him treatments he may not wish for. Against this backdrop it is particularly challenging for therapists to create contexts that have genuine therapeutic potential. In attempting to create such contexts, our intention is to enter our meetings with families with a stance of non-judgemental *curiosity* (Cecchin 1987) and to create an atmosphere marked by mutual listening and respect, which invites reflection and the emergence of new understandings and new ways of going on (Fredman 2007).

Thus, in preparing to meet with Pallab and his family, it was important for us to reflect on how our pre-understandings, based on our conversations with the referring MDT, were influencing us. We have a lot of respect for our colleagues and knew that their intentions were to work with Pallab to secure his lasting health and his own and others' safety. We were sympathetic to their frustration at finding that the family's involvement was limiting their effectiveness; and we were aware that this pre-understanding and sympathy could influence our way of being with the family. So we also thought about how the family might be anticipating our meeting, aware that they were coming at our request and had not asked for our involvement. Drawing on our experience of talking with many families in similar situations, we thought they might position us as representatives of a hostile institution and anticipate that we would blame and criticise them. We wondered what they would expect from us as a team of white British professionals. Perhaps they would expect us to misunderstand or to pathologise aspects of their culture that were profoundly important to them. We thought they might be conscious of a huge power differential between our institution and themselves. One family we worked with drew our attention to this in a particularly memorable way. The young patient was delaying his progress by focusing exclusively on fighting for discharge. His father advised him, 'Son, when your head is in the mouth of a lion, you pull it out slowly.' Holding these ideas about the family's perspective in mind helped us to approach our meeting with them in a stance of appreciation and genuine curiosity.

The questioning therapist and the reflecting team

The systemic theory briefly described above is enacted in the methods used in our practice. The reader will be familiar with the use of 'teams' in family therapy. Team-working has evolved over time and today there are a number of models in use. Our own practice involves the use of the *Reflecting Team* (Andersen 1987) in which a single therapist talks with the family while the 'team' of colleagues listens. At one or more point/s during the session the therapist and family take a break in their talking and quietly listen while the team members talk to each other, in front of the family, about what they have been listening to. One-way screens are commonly used in this approach, with the team entering the therapy room to share their reflections. Our own preference, following feedback from families, is for the team to be in the room throughout the session, sitting apart from the family and therapist. Ideally the team will consist of two or three therapists, but with limited resources our practice more commonly involves a 'team' of just one. In this situation the therapist joins her colleague at intervals to conduct a reflecting team conversation and then rejoins the family to continue talking with them.

Whilst talking with the family the therapist engages in a process of *circular questioning*, a form of questioning intended to generate information about *relationships* – relationships between people; between people and contexts; and between meaning and action (Tomm 1984). In one episode with the Kapoor family, for instance, I asked Pallab, 'If something happened to prevent your parents bringing in food for you, who do you think would miss that most?' Pallab replied that he would miss it as he liked his mother's cooking much more than the hospital food but that he thought his mother would miss it too. I asked Mr Kapoor if he agreed with this and when he said he did, I asked what might make it so important for his wife. Mrs Kapoor interrupted to declare passionately, 'I would not be able to hold my head up anywhere if I didn't do it.' As I asked who would judge Mrs Kapoor and what would be behind their judgements, the family told me that their extended family and community would disapprove; and that, in their culture, when a relative is 'ill in hospital' the family has an absolute *obligation* to look after them. In addition both parents spoke of *wanting* to provide food as a way of maintaining the bond with their son which they felt was threatened by the nature of their separation. Pallab spoke indignantly of clinicians' attempts to stop his parents bringing in food and, he assumed, to 'get me away' from the family. Thus we came to understand a little more about the relationship between Pallab and his parents, mediated through food. We saw how the significant system included the extended family and community and we heard how, in the context of their culture, having a relative in hospital had a particular meaning for the family, requiring particular actions.

The reflecting team gives the family the unusual opportunity to listen to their own experiences, positions and dilemmas reflected back to them in the 'third person'. Reflecting team members speak respectfully about what they have heard, staying close to the language used by the family. They are valuing of multiple perspectives and don't seek premature resolution of difference. They may also introduce new ideas (connected to what the family has been talking about), which they 'float lightly' (Fredman 2006, p.7) using tentative, speculative language. And the family, just listening and not being required to respond, is in a position to contemplate these new ideas rather than to immediately accept or reject them. The presence of the team can also help maintain therapeutic boundaries by noticing the current position of the therapist in relation to the family (too close or too distant) and introducing alternative positions in their reflections.

Thus, in the episode with Pallab's family described above, the reflecting team spoke of their admiration for the parents' commitment to doing what was right, their loyalty to their culture and their protection of the bond with their son in extraordinarily difficult circumstances; and they noted how Pallab seemed to share and support his parents' commitments. They wondered whether there were any costs to such commitment for the parents, who had many other responsibilities too. They wondered if Pallab ever found himself in a predicament and whether loyalty to his family and love of his mother's food ever conflicted with the need to show himself in particular ways in the hospital in order to gain his doctors' approval. One team member said that the family's conversation had reminded her of the difference between cultures that valued independence and those that valued interdependence. Another said she had found herself wondering about the perspective of Pallab's MDT. She wondered if they had a similar idea about the importance of food in relationships and whether Pallab sharing food with the 'hospital community' and developing his own skills in cooking might be seen as part of his 'treatment'. She wasn't sure but she wondered if that would put the family in an impossible dilemma in that helping Pallab to progress through hospital might mean looking after him *less*.

When I returned to talking to the family, Mr and Mrs Kapoor spoke of their relief at feeling 'understood' and their sense of battling with the hospital constantly to do the right thing for their son. Mrs Kapoor spoke of what her attentions to her son were 'costing her' (a cost she was willing to pay) and Mr Kapoor said he had not understood before that they might *help* Pallab by encouraging him to eat and cook in the hospital. Pallab anxiously affirmed the importance of his family and his *need* for them to bring him food.

THE THERAPY UNFOLDS

I have referred above to elements of our work with the Kapoor family, in relation to aspects of theory and method. I will summarise below how the therapy unfolded.

Respecting family boundaries

Elizur (1994) highlights how families in contact with agencies of social control are likely to experience multiple breaching of family boundaries, in which their relationships are scrutinised and critiqued. These processes can lead families to strenuously resist further intrusion or to act in provocative ways to test how their boundaries will be respected. Mindful of this, in meeting with the Kapoor family we didn't assume we had their permission to talk about family relationships. We respected the family's boundary until they led us into talk of their relationships. We asked what was most pressing for them and they spoke about their difficult relationship with the hospital, which they perceived as punitive of Pallab and rejecting of his parents. It has often been our experience that we need to attend to issues of relationships and boundaries between the hospital and the family before we can begin to talk about family relationships; and with some families this work can be enough to free the patient to engage more rewardingly with other aspects of the treatment programme.

The boundary of care

For the Kapoor family the boundary conflict between themselves and the hospital was being enacted through the medium of physical care – feeding and laundry. Further conversations about food followed the extract given above and we also began talking with Pallab's MDT about what we were learning from the family about the meaning of bringing food. Pallab's primary nurse joined us for a family meeting in which we negotiated a way forward. The nurse showed respect for the value of the family's bringing food and offered better facilities for sharing food on the ward during their visits; and Mr and Mrs Kapoor recognised the value of Pallab becoming more involved in the ward community and in food preparation and agreed only to bring food twice a week. They planned how they would explain to their community that this was a way of helping their son's treatment and they encouraged a reluctant Pallab to assume his responsibilities on the ward. Some time later the primary nurse, who was by now enthusiastically allied with Mrs Kapoor, suggested on her own initiative that Mrs Kapoor could help Pallab learn to do his own laundry by doing it with him on the ward. Mrs Kapoor agreed, but the suggestion provoked a strong reaction from Pallab. He said he did not need his mother to teach him to use a washing machine and was quite capable of doing it himself.

Thus Pallab began to draw a new boundary in his relationship with his mother and to assert his adult authority.

Talking of boundaries

In family therapy we invited Pallab to strengthen this boundary by speaking about why it was important to him to refuse his mother's offer to teach him to do his washing. He spoke about how humiliating it would be for his peers to witness his mother's involvement in his life on the ward and about his wish to appear as an independent man in their eyes. From this position he became able to talk about similar conflicts he had experienced earlier in his life such as when he was a teenager straddling two cultures, trying to follow family traditions at home while struggling to be accepted by his peers at school. As this latter imperative became stronger he started drinking and using cannabis as a way of belonging to his peer group. For Pallab the attempt to maintain a rigid boundary between his identities at home and in the outside world became an impossible burden.

Regrets and moral boundaries

In our early sessions with the family Mr Kapoor spoke at length about how, as parents, they had done everything to give their children a good upbringing; and how he could think of nothing in family life that could explain what had happened to Pallab. We accepted this and expressed appreciation of the family's admirable efforts and intentions. It took my breath away when, some way into our work, Mr Kapoor, unprompted, said quietly, 'I have so many regrets.' Over the following sessions he began to speak of how, preoccupied with working to support the family, he had paid insufficient attention to his son. Often tired and stressed, he had been quick to criticise; and wanting his son to do well he had expected too much of him, pushed him too hard. Pallab listened with rapt attention. Pallab went on to speak of his own regrets and the family began to talk, for the first time, about his offence and what it meant to each of them. Mrs Kapoor wept as she and her husband spoke about the family's shame and horror that their son had seriously injured a good and innocent neighbour, contrary to everything they stood for as a family. They spoke of their own feelings of guilt that they had not recognised how ill their son had become and had not acted to prevent what had happened. The parents' stating of the family's moral boundary and their obvious distress clearly moved Pallab. Previously he had seemed to view the moral boundary as drawn by hostile institutions and spoke of 'regret' in a superficial, placatory way. Now he began to speak of his offence as a breach of his own and his family's moral boundaries and in the painfulness of this realisation he and his parents were able to join in a resolution that nothing like this should ever happen again. By this point the intentions of the family and the institution had merged and the rigid boundary between them had become sufficiently flexible for Pallab to work with his team with his parents' support. The boundaries within the family had also begun to move towards a new position, in which Pallab could belong while also developing adult autonomy and authority.

CONCLUSION

In this chapter I have offered a small picture of what a systemic family therapy approach might bring to working with boundaries in a forensic mental health setting. I have suggested the importance of considering boundary issues between the family and the institution as well as within the family. And I have presented how we attempt to create therapeutic contexts in family therapy in this challenging setting by being mindful of what we each bring to the encounter and by respecting the family's boundaries.

REFERENCES

Andersen, T. (1987) 'The reflecting team: dialogue and meta-dialogue in clinical work.' *Family Process 26*, 415–428.

Boscolo, L., Cecchin, G, Hoffman, L. and Penn, P. (1987) *Milan Systemic Family Therapy*. New York: Basic Books.

Cecchin, G. (1987) 'Hypothesising, circularity and neutrality revisited: an invitation to curiosity.' *Family Process 26*, 405–413.

Davies, B and Harre, R. (1990) 'Positioning: the discursive production of selves.' *Journal for the Theory of Social Behaviour 20*, 43–64.

Elizur, Y. (1994) 'Working with families in institutions for juvenile offenders: an eco-systemic model for the development of family involvement.' *Human Systems Journal 5*, 3–4, 253–266.

Fredman, G. (2006) 'Working systemically with intellectual disabilities: why not?' In S. Baum and H. Lynggaard (eds) *Intellectual Disabilities: A Systemic Approach*. London: Karnac.

Fredman, G. (2007) 'Preparing Ourselves for the Therapeutic Relationship: Revisiting "Hypothesising Revisited".' *Human Systems Journal 18*, 44–59.

Griffith, J.L. and Elliott Griffith, M. (1994) *The Body Speaks: Therapeutic Dialogues for Mind-Body Problems*. New York: Basic Books.

Jones, E. (1993) *Family Systems Therapy*. Chichester: Wiley-Blackwell.

McNamee, S. and Gergen, K. (1992) *Therapy as Social Construction*. Newbury Park, CA: Sage.

Minuchin, S. (1974) *Families and Family Therapy*. London: Tavistock Publications.

Tomm, K. (1984) 'One Perspective on the Milan Approach: Part 1. Overview of development, theory and practice.' *Journal of Marital and Family Therapy 10*, 2, 113–125.

Watzlawick, P., Beavin Bavelas, J. and Jackson, D. (1967) *Pragmatics of Human Communication*. London and New York: W.W. Norton & Company.

Chapter 9

BOUNDARIES IN FORENSIC MENTAL HEALTH NURSING: SET IN STONE OR SHIFTING SANDS?

Gillian Kelly and Emma Wadey

Overview

Issues surrounding boundaries within forensic mental health services are often a major challenge for all professionals. Within these settings patients' uncontained and unresolved feelings frequently manifest in complex and clinically challenging behaviours, such as boundary testing, rule breaking, threats and violence. Through these behaviours, unprocessed emotions are acted out and/or projected into clinicians who are then required to maintain therapeutic boundaries and enforce limits whilst they are also struggling to process a range of powerful emotions such as fear, frustration, humiliation and anger, to name but a few. Left unaddressed, this dynamic can create a massive sense of physical and psychological insecurity in clinicians, patients and the wider organisation. In turn the setting and maintenance of boundaries becomes even more difficult. Boundaries can start to drift and a slippery slope from boundary crossings to major violations can occur.

This chapter will explore how the uniqueness of the nurse's task can further complicate the already challenging work of boundary maintenance within forensic inpatient settings. We will also describe key requirements for nurses working in secure settings and make recommendations as to the guiding principles for the maintenance of effective professional and therapeutic boundaries.

A case example and discussion will be used to explore and highlight some of the themes discussed. Although drawn from an amalgam of clinical experiences, all clinical examples used are fictitious to ensure confidentiality.

BOUNDARIES AND THE FORENSIC MENTAL HEALTH NURSE'S TASK

The Oxford Dictionary (2011) defines a boundary as 'a line which marks the limits…'. Although this simplistic definition may be helpful for initiating thinking about boundaries, it does not reflect the complex task of setting and maintaining professional and therapeutic boundaries within nursing.

The mental health nurse's main therapeutic tool is the nurse–patient relationship, through which the nurse helps the patient to make therapeutic gains (Aiyegbusi 2004). It is well documented that boundaries have an important containing function and can help to protect the patient and clinician as well as protect and preserve the therapeutic relationship (Brown and Sobart 2008). With this in mind it is easy to see how crucial boundaries are in nursing and how the boundaries which encompass the nurse–patient relationship are central not only to the nurse's task but also to the quality, safety and effectiveness of the relationship.

The forensic setting and the nature of patients' offending bring additional challenges for the nurse, who as a result may be tested and stretched beyond conventional limits. In our experience the maintenance of boundaries in forensic nursing is more akin to trying to negotiate a path through shifting sands rather than one road set in stone. There are very few clear lines that mark the limits. The reason for this becomes apparent when you consider not only the prolonged periods of interpersonal contact nurses have with patients who present with complex and clinically challenging behaviours, but also the variety, intensity and unpredictability of tasks nurses are expected to undertake. Furthermore, the majority of the nurse's work takes place within the environmental context of a ward, which in addition to being the setting for psychiatric treatment is also the patient's domestic and social environment. This multifunctional environment is fertile ground for the development of many boundary issues.

Within one span of duty, a nurse can easily be undertaking a number of activities with patients that on their own raise multiple boundary issues and collectively even more so. Nurses are required to provide one-to-one support, sometimes several times a day or for several hours at a time. Nursing on a ward means you do not have the inbuilt containment provided by the therapeutic hour or the extra thinking space that offices away from the clinical environment can facilitate.

Nurses often find themselves having to move from task to task without spaces in between to stop and reflect. For instance, a nurse may be required to observe a patient whilst bathing and using the toilet as well as undertake intimate physical health care or an examination. Next a nurse may engage in a communal meal or be required to facilitate and engage in social activities with patients such as ward parties or playing board games. Numerous boundary issues can arise in relation to any of these tasks, which can feel unpredictable for nurses. In addition, the conflicting boundary positions needed for each task are often difficult to negotiate. For example, the boundaries involved in observing a patient in the bath are very different from those needed at a communal meal or ward party. The patient's responses to the different boundaries can also further challenge the nurse. For instance, the patient may take the intimate experience of being seen naked in the bath or the touch involved in a health care procedure as the baseline for boundaries surrounding the relationship. The patient may then find it difficult to understand why wearing revealing clothing or trying to hug a nurse at the ward party may not be appropriate, especially given the previous levels of intimacy, and as a result become confused, upset and angry with the nurse.

The forensic setting brings an additional layer of complexity for nurses. A key component of this is the long-term nature of the therapeutic relationship in forensic settings. Patients may be in hospital for several years, which increases the intensity of relationships between patients and nurses as well as the risk of dependency. An example of how this level of familiarity manifests is the way that patients frequently describe and behave as if nurses are their extended or only family. This 'as if' process is likely to be compounded or caused by complex transference and counter-transference processes that bring a minefield of boundary dilemmas. For instance, if a nurse is thought of or referred to as mother, father, auntie or uncle it can set up an unhealthy, unboundaried dynamic that has the potential to be very damaging for both the patient and nurse.

The forensic nurse at times will have to set limits in the face of threatening, intimidating, sexualized and violent behaviours and, when necessary, physically restrain a patient to ensure their safety and that of the patient and others. Maintaining the boundaries of the therapeutic relationship, especially boundaries around touch, when under certain circumstances you may have no choice but to physically restrain a patient, is very challenging. This becomes extremely complicated when you consider the potential for traumatic experiences to get re-enacted through restraint, and that for some patients behaving in a way that forces nurses into this type of re-enactment may be their only means of communicating distress.

Within the forensic setting there is also the risk that boundaries become punitive, degrading and anti-therapeutic, particularly when a balanced or holistic stance could be more difficult to maintain. This is particularly true in relation to risk management where the temptation and/or need to control all risk, and its associated anxiety, by limiting the patient's access to risk items can prevent the use of therapeutic risk-taking and limit progress. For instance, managing an individual's risk to self by completely stripping their bedroom of all items with the potential for harm can be experienced and sometimes used in a punitive way. The intervention becomes counter-therapeutic, serving to increase rather than decrease risk. A battle of wills can emerge and the patients may respond by resorting to more creative and sometimes more lethal methods of harming themselves.

However, it is important to remember that all the components of nursing described above also make nursing exceptional. Nurses are privileged to be able to work with patients in these ways and have the opportunity to use these experiences not only to role-model professional and therapeutic boundaries, which many patients may have lacked in their early life experiences, but also to build on the mental health nurse's main therapeutic tool: the nurse–patient relationship.

BOUNDARY PHENOMENA

In our experience there are two main types of boundary phenomena that repeatedly occur in interactions with patients within forensic mental health settings. These are insidious boundary testing and high-impact boundary testing.

Insidious boundary testing occurs over time with a gradual chipping away of the boundary during everyday interactions, such as over a cup of tea. During these types of interactions patients may ask the nurse personal questions and over time the nurse may gradually disclose more and more personal information and may even become over-involved with the patient. This insidious boundary testing can go unnoticed and the new ways of relating can become the accepted 'norm' until things gradually spiral out of control.

High-impact boundary testing, on the other hand, is much more immediate and unpredictable. This type of boundary testing requires the maintenance of boundaries or setting of limits in the face of threats, intimidation or even violence. In these situations there is little, if any, time to think and reflect. Action is often required immediately to ensure the safety of both the patient and others. These types of phenomena may also occur as a result of setting a boundary or limit which can evoke an explosive response from the patient. The immediacy and lack of space to think associated with this type of boundary testing can increase the risk of boundary crossings. For instance, a punitive response to threatening behaviour is more likely if you have no time to process the fact that you have been threatened, and feel frightened, angry or defensive.

In these situations the challenge for the nurse is to process powerful emotions whilst simultaneously having to act or, as Aiyegbusi puts, it 'to think under fire' (Aiyegbusi 2002, p.113).

Boundary phenomena can also emanate from professionals, including nurses. For example, our own personal history can affect our ability to set and maintain boundaries. This may include one's personal reasons for choosing to work in a helping profession; as well as individual's current and past experiences, which, similarly to patients, can include unresolved trauma. Other important factors that can impact on an individual's ability to set and maintain professional boundaries include interpersonal skills, the extent of knowledge and experience of the patient group and care setting, cultural values and beliefs, and whether or not they have the spaces and capacity to reflect.

The two ways boundary phenomena tend to manifest in relation to nursing is either a failure to maintain boundaries pertaining to one's professional role or a failure to maintain therapeutic limits and boundaries in relation to the planned care and treatment of patients. These two areas have significant overlap as professional boundaries relating to role may also be therapeutic. For example, limiting the amount or type of personal disclosures made by a nurse is both a professional as well as a therapeutic boundary.

Although it may be tempting to try and understand boundary phenomena as emanating either from staff or patients, the picture is usually more complex. This is especially true when we begin to think about boundaries from an organisational perspective.

In our experience, it is not uncommon for the boundary phenomena from patients and nurses to become enmeshed and then further compounded by organisational issues. For example, a boundary issue may arise when a nurse responds to a patient's challenging behaviour in an unprofessional way. Exploration of this incident may, in addition to identifying problems relating to the conduct of the individual nurse, uncover numerous systemic issues, such as:

- failure to fully address previous incidents involving the patient
- failure to fully address previous incidents involving nurses' and/or other professionals' conduct in relation to the patient
- inadequate formulation, care planning and care delivery
- poor multi-disciplinary working
- a lack of opportunities or systems for effective clinical supervision and reflective practice
- poor professional and clinical leadership

- absence of relevant training and development opportunities
- a culture of blame that focuses exclusively on the individual, ignoring the wider clinical and organisational context.

It is our view that it is crucial to take a whole systems perspective on boundaries rather than just focus on individuals. Failure to explore the wider picture, including boundaries relating to the organisation and its systems, will increase the risk of a repetitive cycle of boundary violations.

Case example

Kirsty is a 30-year-old woman who suffered regular physical, sexual and emotional abuse from her husband. After being assaulted by her husband and whilst under the influence of drugs and alcohol, which they both abused regularly, Kirsty killed her husband by stabbing him with a knife. She was sentenced to prison. However, after becoming depressed and suicidal, Kirsty was transferred to a secure mental health hospital for assessment.

Once admitted to hospital Kirsty spent considerable periods of time being nursed on one-to-one observations, during which nurses engaged Kirsty in conversation, day-to-day living tasks and other therapeutic activities. Kirsty found one-to-one observations very intrusive apart from when Pauline, her primary nurse, undertook them. As a result, whenever Pauline was on duty she undertook Kirsty's one-to-one observations for several hours during her span of duty. This was also encouraged by most of Pauline's nursing colleagues, who found it difficult to be with Kirsty.

Kirsty would talk to Pauline about her traumatic experiences with her husband and go over and over the details of her index offence. She began to express that only Pauline understood her and she refused to engage with other members of the nursing and clinical team. Kirsty became very explosive and argumentative with the other nurses on the ward. All Kirsty's requests began to be channelled through Pauline, who was becoming increasing exhausted and overwhelmed in trying to meet Kirsty's needs. Pauline began buying food and gifts for Kirsty, which was not permitted under the hospital's policies.

When challenged by her peers, Pauline became angry and told Kirsty that she was no longer able to buy things for her because her colleagues were complaining. In turn, Kirsty became angry and upset and began assaulting the other nurses for stopping Pauline bringing her food and gifts. The nurses and wider clinical team became angry and frustrated with Pauline and blamed her for their difficulties with Kirsty. Ostracised from her peers, Pauline began to confide more and more in Kirsty, sharing personal information with her about her own relationship difficulties both at work and at home.

Several weeks later, during a one-to-one session, Kirsty attempted to strangle Pauline, causing her serious injuries. When the clinical team asked Kirsty why she tried to strangle Pauline, Kirsty reported that she was overwhelmed and felt trapped in a relationship with Pauline, who she felt was offloading her own problems onto her just like her husband used to do.

Pauline, who made a full recovery from her physical injuries, was subject to a formal investigation and issued with a final written warning for her inappropriate conduct. She was moved to an alternative ward. She was also referred to occupational health and offered staff support. However, she was left feeling unsupported and angry.

Subsequently, Kirsty was allocated a new primary nurse who also became quite overwhelmed by her and a similar scenario emerged, which again led to Kirsty's primary nurse being moved to another ward.

Discussion

The case described highlights how boundary phenomena can escalate and how easily patient, staff and organisational issues become enmeshed and entangled. Kirsty's intense pattern of relating and associated risks get re-enacted in her relationships with the nurses on the ward, especially her primary nurse, who becomes overwhelmed. Insidious boundary phenomena is evident as Kirsty's pattern of relating gradually pulls her primary nurse out of role; and without the support of her colleagues Pauline gradually spends more and more time with Kirsty, until she feels exhausted and overwhelmed and begins breaking more boundaries by bringing Kirsty food and toiletries and sharing personal information, in a desperate attempt to meet Kirsty's and her own needs. The situation quickly escalates to high-impact boundary testing as Kirsty assaults staff and finally tries to strangle Pauline. Rather than make sense of the re-enactment the nurses find themselves in, the organisational systems require a formal investigation which focuses on the individual. As such, one person is seen as the problem and moved, while the splitting dynamics in the team as well as the patient's pathology do not get processed and addressed. The failure to look more systemically and holistically results in the scenario re-occurring and the cycle continuing.

REQUIREMENTS FOR NURSES

Nurses, and in particular health care assistants, may have had limited or even no previous experience within mental health or forensic settings. Despite this and the complexities of the nursing task, there continues to be a lack of training and skills development in relation to boundaries. Nurses are also the least likely to have received advanced training to help them in their work, and are the least likely of the multi-professional team to have adequate access to supervision and support. These issues are compounded by the fact there is limited context-specific written guidance on boundaries available for nurses.

Within any mental health setting, but particularly within a secure forensic setting, the testing and stretching of therapeutic boundaries is to be expected and can be an important indicator in assessing the treatment needs of patients. Therefore, a proactive and open culture needs to exist to support and assist both nurses and patients in navigating through the complex boundary dilemmas on a daily basis.

Even when boundaries are defined and guidelines provided, their complexity or the likelihood of them being broken does not simply disappear, as even clearly defined boundaries are regularly transgressed by both professionals and the patients in their care. In addition, just having or knowing a boundary, however concrete, is not always enough to ensure it is maintained.

It is essential for all nurses to be aware of the potential for boundary drift, crossings and violations as well as the dilemmas they will face within clinical practice. They must be supported to develop strategies for responding to boundary situations effectively. They need to be aware of the link between patients' pathologies, histories, presenting behaviours and the effect these have on boundary setting and maintenance with that individual. It is vital that nurses have an awareness of factors that may influence one's ability to set and maintain boundaries, such as knowledge of transference and counter-transference processes (Aiyegbusi 2002; Temple 1996), personal valency (Bion 1961), personal factors that increase the risk of boundary violations and the importance of accessing spaces for thought and reflection.

As much as individual nurses are accountable for their own practice, nurses also have collective responsibility for their colleagues. If a nurse is at risk from 'sliding down the slippery slope of boundary crossings to violations', other nurses are likely to be aware that something is not right and are perfectly placed to intervene by talking to that person and seeking out a senior colleague or manager as required.

BOUNDARIES WORKSHOP

Within our work organisation, one of the ways we have tried to address boundary issues is through the development of a workshop aimed at helping nurses set and maintain therapeutic boundaries with patients in secure settings. The workshop is specifically aimed at addressing the emotionality involved in boundary setting as well as giving advice on day-to-day practice issues. To achieve this we have found it helpful to incorporate aspects of forensic psychotherapy and psychoanalytical concepts with nursing practice.

More specifically the workshop addresses:

- what is a boundary

- why boundaries are important, and guiding principles for boundary setting and maintenance

- boundaries in secure care, including: linking patients' mental health problems, diagnoses, histories, offending and presenting behaviours to boundary issues

- factors influencing professionals' boundaries, including personal risk factors and warning signs

- responding to boundary crossings and violations, including giving and receiving feedback

- systemic considerations, including the multi-disciplinary team and roles

- prevention of serious incidents: exploring structures that support effective boundary setting

- scenarios (on DVD) and subsequent group discussion

- common boundary dilemmas and workplace experiences through discussion

- useful reading and tools, including *The Nursing Boundary Index*.

(Pilette, Berck and Achber 1995)

In day-to-day practice the workshop is underpinned by clinical supervision and reflective forums. The workshop provides participants with a basic clinical framework for reflecting upon and managing professional and therapeutic boundaries in secure settings, whilst clinical supervision and reflective forums provide practitioners and teams with spaces to utilise the framework. This approach aims to help facilitate continuous learning.

In terms of measuring the effectiveness of the workshop we have undertaken regular reviews of the workshop feedback questionnaires and have also undertaken an audit of nurses' and patients' perspectives on boundaries (Wadey 2011). The audit included obtaining views on what constitutes a boundary being transgressed and what helps support the maintenance of boundaries in day-to-day practice. This data, alongside anecdotal evidence and an informal review of incidents, indicates that the workshop is effective in better equipping nurses to manage boundaries as well as reducing boundary incidents. However, a more detailed evaluation of the workshop would be helpful, as well as more research in relation to boundaries and the efficacy of training in reducing boundary breaking.

CONCLUSION

The uniqueness of the nursing task and the challenging environment of a secure setting in combination with a clinically complex patient group provide fertile ground for conflict and dilemmas in the effective maintenance of professional and therapeutic boundaries.

Although it is widely acknowledged that boundary drift, crossings and violations are common phenomena, there has been a paucity of training opportunities or specifically identified support for nursing staff to manage them.

Services need to find ways to support and educate nurses in relation to setting and maintaining boundaries. Within our services a workshop to explore the complexities for therapeutic boundary setting and maintenance was developed to provide a basic clinical framework and reflective forum to explore and support the management of boundaries in day-to-day practice as well as help reduce the occurrence of boundary breaking. The workshop has been underpinned by clinical supervision and reflective practice forums.

However, further work needs to be done on developing a more proactive and open culture within organisational structures whereby the likelihood for boundary transgressions is acknowledged but dealt with in a consistent, transparent and supportive way, and where collective responsibility for their maintenance is the norm.

REFERENCES

Aiyegbusi, A. (2002) 'Thinking Under Fire: The Challenge for Forensic Mental Health Nurses Working with Women in Secure Care.' In N. Jeffcote and T. Watson (eds) (2004) *Working Therapeutically with Women in Secure Settings*. London: Jessica Kingsley Publishers.

Aiyegbusi, A. (2004) 'Forensic Mental Health Nursing: Care with Security in Mind.' In F. Pfäfflin and G. Adshead (eds) *A Matter of Security: The Application of Attachment Theory to Forensic Psychiatry and Psychotherapy*. London: Jessica Kingsley Publishers.

Bion, W.R. (1961) *Experiences in groups and other papers*. London: Tavistock Publications. Reprinted: Routledge 1989.

Brown, R. and Sobart, K. (2008) *Understanding Boundaries and Containment in Clinical Practice.* London: Karnac Books.

Oxford Dictionary (2011) Available at www.oxforddictionaries.com/definition/boundary, accessed on 27 February 2012.

Pilette, P., Berck, C. and Achber, L. (1995) 'Therapeutic management.' *Journal of Psychosocial Nursing and Mental Health Services 33*, 1, 40–47.

Temple, N. (1996) 'Transference and Countertransference – General and Forensic Aspects.' In C. Cordess and M. Cox *Forensic Psychotherapy: Crime, Psychodynamics and the Offender Patient. Volume 1: Mainly Theory.* London: Jessica Kingley Publishers.

Wadey, E. (2011) 'Boundaries in secure care: A comparative audit of nursing and patient perceptions.' Unpublished.

Chapter 10

BOUNDARIES AND DESIRE IN FORENSIC MENTAL HEALTH NURSING

Cindy Peternelj-Taylor

We desire nothing so much as what we ought not to have.

Publilius Syrus, c.100 BC

Overview

Desire is not a word that we typically associate with the therapeutic nurse–client relationship, rather it is one that is generally reserved for the intimacy between lovers. And while it is recognized that the potential for boundary violations exists in all relationships, it is the intensity of the forensic milieu that contributes to the immediacy of complicated relationships. Forensic mental health nurses are clearly influenced by the clientele with whom they work and the organizational context in which they find themselves; thus the impact of the physical and interpersonal climate on therapeutic relationships cannot be ignored (Peternelj-Taylor 1998, 2003). When forensic mental health nurses negate their roles in establishing and maintaining therapeutic boundaries, and use their relationships with clients to meet their personal needs, they are at risk of over-involvement. In practice, over-involvement frequently leads to sexual boundary violations (Gutheil and Brodsky 2008).

In this chapter, the phenomenon of sexual boundary violations within the context of the forensic milieu will be examined. Specific issues and dilemmas unique to the manifestation of sexual boundary violations by forensic mental health nurses will be explored and illustrated with reference to clinical scenarios and contemporary literature. Unfortunately, sexual boundary violations are a distressing reality of clinical practice with forensic clients; one that places forensic mental health nurses at increased risk of transgressing treatment boundaries (Faulkner and Regehr 2011; Peternelj-Taylor 1998, 2003; Thomas-Peter and Garrett 2000). It is hoped that through this exploration into sexual boundary violations, forensic mental health nurses will be in a better position to work therapeutically with this risk.

SCOPE OF SEXUAL BOUNDARY VIOLATIONS IN THE FORENSIC MILIEU

In recent years there has been increased attention paid to the topic of boundary violations in therapeutic nurse–client relationships, leading some authors to conclude that sexual boundary violations in forensic mental health settings should be conceptualized as an occupational hazard and not simply a social and professional taboo (Love and Heber 2002; Peternelj-Taylor 1998, 2002; Schafer and Peternelj-Taylor 2003). However, to date there has been little nursing research published regarding sexual boundary violations in the forensic mental health nursing literature. It is as though discussions surrounding sexual boundary violations in the forensic milieu are "too hot to handle" (Fronek *et al.* 2009), despite the fact that such violations represent grave clinical and security issues – issues that have a profound impact on the whole organization in which they occur (Thomas-Peter and Garrett 2000). And while most forensic mental health nurses would consider sexual boundary violations as a flagrant abuse of their power within the nurse–client relationship, the phenomenon remains poorly understood. Sexual boundary violations are defined by Celenza (2007) as "any kind of physical contact occurring in the context of a therapeutic relationship for the purpose of erotic pleasure" (p.5). The Council for Healthcare Regulatory Excellence (CHRE 2008), states "…a breach of sexual boundaries occurs when a healthcare professional displays sexualized behaviour towards a patient or carer. Sexualized behaviour is defined as acts, words or behaviour designed or intended to arouse or gratify sexual impulses or desires" (p.14). Hugging, hand-holding, kissing, petting, oral sex, and intercourse have been reported (Bachmann *et al.* 2000; Thomas-Peter and Garrett 2000).

Given the sensitive nature of sexual boundary violations in forensic mental health settings, determining the exact extent of the problem is particularly challenging. Much of what is known about sexual boundary violations remains largely circumstantial. Forensic organizations are generally averse to public discourse surrounding this clinical problem (Evershed 2011), so much so that forensic mental health staff who engage in sexual boundary violations are rarely reported to their licensing or regulatory bodies. Instead, nurses resign under the threat of an investigation, and move out of the jurisdiction (Peternelj-Taylor 2003).

Anecdotal wisdom would suggest, however, that every nurse who has ever worked in a forensic mental health setting knows of at least one case of a sexual boundary violation, as illustrated in the words of an experienced forensic mental health nurse:

> I have seen many staff members actually leave their jobs to be with offenders; in my career at least a dozen. One day I actually stopped counting because there were so many.[1]

Finding actual statistics on sexual boundary violations within forensic mental health nursing is particularly challenging. What is known about sexual boundary violations has generally been borrowed from other disciplines. Thomas-Peter and Garrett (2000) have suggested, however, that perpetrators of sexual boundary violations in forensic settings are predominantly female, whereas in general psychiatric units the perpetrators are predominantly male. This begs the question, is gender truly a factor in sexual boundary violations in forensic mental health settings? Or is it simply that the clientele in forensic settings is predominantly male and the forensic mental health nurses predominantly female?

FACTORS INFLUENCING SEXUAL BOUNDARY VIOLATIONS

Sexual misconduct is not a phenomenon unique to forensic mental health nursing. However, forensic mental health nurses appear to be at increased risk for transgressing sexual boundaries, due to a combination of factors, including limited education and training regarding boundary violations, client and nurse vulnerability, and the nature of the nurse–client relationship.

Education and training

It is normal for health professionals to feel attracted to their clients, yet many professional groups, including nurses, only receive token education related to sexual boundaries in their basic education programs, and very little education following graduation (Fronek et al. 2009). Feelings of sexual attraction are frequently accompanied by guilt, shame and confusion, particularly among inexperienced nurses, who in turn respond with avoidance, denial, or punitive

---

1   Unpublished research data from the author's study entitled "The Lived Experience of Engagement with Forensic Patients in Secure Environments."

limit setting (Gutheil and Brodsky 2008). Clearly the importance of primary prevention is critical given the universality of sexual attraction and how easily boundaries can be crossed (Bachmann *et al.* 2000). Unfortunately, education that nurses may have received on the subject of sexual boundary violations is rarely discussed in relation to the ongoing development of the therapeutic alliance, or common relationship issues such as transference, counter transference or resistance.

Client vulnerability

By virtue of their status as *forensic* clients, as a group they are clearly vulnerable. They are also often uncertain about the nature of boundaries and how transgressions might be addressed. Such uncertainty contributes further to their vulnerability (Schafer and Peternelj-Taylor 2003). However, this vulnerability is rarely recognized; instead, forensic clients are conceptualized in terms of the threat they pose to nurses. Clients are seen as perpetrators, nurses as victims. And although the responsibility for establishing and maintaining professional boundaries rests with the forensic mental health nurse, Faulkner and Regehr (2011) argue that many forensic clients are skilled at manipulation and exploiting situations for their personal gain, thus contributing to a blurring of the lines of responsibility when sexual violations do occur. Although such a characterization may be true for some clients, particularly those with psychopathic disorder (Thomas-Peter and Garrett, 2000), it is always the professional's responsibility to establish, monitor and manage the boundaries of the relationship (Celenza 2007).

Nurse vulnerability

Therapy issues with forensic clients can be particularly complex, and novice and seasoned forensic nurses alike experience challenges in the provision of safe and professional care. The seductive pull of helping, coupled with the dual obligation of providing custody and caring, can contribute to nurse vulnerability regarding management of therapeutic boundaries. Many forensic clients are particularly powerful, dominant, intimidating, needy, charming, good-looking and attentive. Gutheil and Brodsky (2008) conclude that even the most ethical among us can be tested by the manipulative behaviors of the clients in our care. Nurses who are particularly at risk for transgressing boundaries are nurses who: 1) have difficulties differentiating the professional relationship from a social relationship; and 2) those who strive to have their needs met through their relationships with clients (Pilette, Berck and Achber 1995). Nurses suffer the same frailties as other human beings. Often they are most vulnerable during times when they are experiencing major life stressors such as illness, changing life circumstances, relationship problems, bereavement, or personal caregiving responsibilities (Faulkner and Regehr 2011; Norris, Gutheil and Strasburger 2003). Such vulnerabilities, can lead to role reversal and inappropriate self-disclosure on the part of the nurse.

Therapists, including forensic nurses, who engage in sexual boundary violations generally fall into one of three categories: narcissistic psychopaths, those who are psychotic, and those who are "lovesick" (Twemlow and Gabbard 1989). And while all three categories of offending therapists can be found in forensic mental health nursing, in the author's personal experience most sexual boundary violations occurring in forensic mental health settings are of the lovesick variety. More recently, Faulkner and Regehr (2011) have concluded that not only are those experiencing personal problems at increased risk of transgressing boundaries to fulfil their personal needs, they are also at risk of being targeted by forensic clients who seek to exploit the relationship for personal gain.

Nature of the nurse–client relationship

When compared to other forensic mental health disciplines, the nurse–client relationship appears somewhat less formal, even though the power imbalance remains the same. In many settings, forensic nurses practice where their clients live, and as such it is not uncommon for them to spend a significant amount of time with their clients, often over days, weeks, months, and in some cases, years. Given the diversity of roles and responsibilities unique to forensic nursing, nurses find themselves engaged in addressing their clients' physical and psychosocial health care needs, administering medications and treatments, engaging them in individual and group activities, and providing for safety and security. And although every activity that the forensic nurse engages in should be for the therapeutic benefit of the client, many forensic nursing activities appear more social, informal or spontaneous in nature, which can be very confusing for the clients (Schafer and Peternelj-Taylor 2003). Love and Heber (2002) have concluded that weekends and evenings can be particularly problematic, as forensic nurses often take part in unstructured client activities, for prolonged periods of time, with limited supervision, leading to spontaneous "small-talk" and to unplanned disclosures on the part of the forensic mental health nurse (Evershed 2011).

Furthermore, engaging in the nurse–client relationship and working with a forensic client on his or her problems can be extremely intimate. Clients share their thoughts, their feelings, their fears, their hopes and their aspirations with nurses who give them undivided attention, who listen empathically, and who provide them with a glimpse of the outside world. It is not uncommon for clients to misinterpret nurses' warmth and concern. Professional experience has shown that clients are ill-prepared for the intimacy that comes with engagement in the therapeutic relationship, yet rarely are they advised of what is considered appropriate or inappropriate behavior with their nurse (Peternelj-Taylor and Schafer 2008). Sexual boundary violations, however, do not simply occur "out the blue" so to speak, rather they are much more likely the result of a number of small deviations from established practice that over time lead to a full-blown boundary violation (Love and Heber 2002; Simon 1995).

Finally, from a regulatory perspective, Fischer, Houchen and Ferguson-Ramos (2008) note that of cases of boundary violations that are reported, two factors are generally present: client vulnerability and prolonged client contact.

RISK MANAGEMENT OF SEXUAL BOUNDARY VIOLATIONS

Prevention of sexual boundary violations in forensic mental health settings requires the open acknowledgement that the potential for abuse exists in all therapeutic relationships. In fact, due to the intensity of the therapeutic relationships that develop within forensic settings, and the insidious nature of sexual boundary violations, Celenza (2007) suggests that rather than ask the question "Why do therapists violate boundaries?", perhaps we should ask instead "Why don't therapists violate boundaries more often?" (p.4). The prevention and management of sexual boundary violations is not something that individual nurses (or other therapists) should shoulder on their own. Rather, the responsibility lies with not only the nurse, but also with the organization in which one is employed, professional bodies, peers and educators (Evershed 2011; Peternelj-Taylor and Schafer 2008).

Self-awareness, self-monitoring and reflective practice

Self-awareness is critical to navigating the therapeutic relationship, avoiding sexual boundary violations, and developing personal risk management strategies. Forensic nurses are not infallible; and like other forensic mental health professionals, they too are vulnerable to transgressing sexual boundaries. It is not uncommon, however, for forensic mental health nurses to seek solace in their belief that "this couldn't happen to me" (Norris *et al.* 2003, p.517). Celenza (2007) suggests that such an omnipotent wish is particularly dangerous. Believing that one is immune to sexual boundary violations only contributes further to one's risk of over-involvement, as those who deny their vulnerability are less likely to recognize warning signs, and less likely to seek consultation.

It is much easier to share feelings of anger, disgust, frustration, even moral outrage, about one's clients with colleagues than it is to share sexual feelings about a client. Forensic nurses should reflect on the following questions:

- How do I set boundaries for my sexual attraction to clients, or for a client's attraction to me? Are there ways in which I am having my intimacy needs met through my clients? (Pennington *et al.* 1993).

- Would I say or do this in front of my supervisor? (Gallop 1998, p.44).

- Is this a behavior or interaction you would want other people to know you had engaged in with a client? (CARNA 2011, p.11).

Such questions used in conjunction with self-assessment tools such as Epstein and Simon's (1990) Exploitation Index, or its modified version, the Nursing Boundary Index (Pilette *et al.* 1995), or most recently the Sexual Boundary Violation Index (Swiggart *et al.* 2008) can assist forensic mental health nurses with reflecting on their practice. As Sarkar (2004) has concluded, all other interventions – education, awareness and supervision – are only effective if one is able to reflect on one's practice. Clearly, being able to critically reflect on one's practice is an essential skill for boundary management (Fronek *et al.* 2009).

Codes of ethics and standards for practice can also inform the forensic mental health nurse regarding ethical practice. And while codes alone cannot promote ethical practice and determine ethical decisions, they can serve as a springboard for further education and dialogue regarding sexual boundary violations (Storch 2007). However, forensic mental health nurses, like all other mental health therapists who engage in sexual boundary violations, know that what they are doing is wrong – they do not need to read it in their code of ethics to know so (Celenza 2007).

Promoting a culture of support: peer debriefing and group prevention strategies

Issues surrounding desire, sexual attraction and forbidden love represent complex clinical issues in the forensic milieu. And while individual forensic mental health nurses are responsible for managing appropriate relationships with their clients, the collective wisdom of a supportive interdisciplinary clinical team, where members are able to openly acknowledge, discuss, and examine their feelings in relation to sexual dilemmas that arise in clinical practice, is an invaluable primary prevention strategy (Fronek, *et al.* 2009; Peternelj-Taylor and Yonge 2003). As such, teams have an essential role to play regarding "harm-minimization" (Evershed 2011). For example, team meetings should be held on a regular basis to discuss issues of sexual attraction and sexual boundary violations before incidents happen, rather than only after they have happened. The use of hypothetical clinical vignettes, case studies and role playing are less threatening to the individual nurse (or other team member) who may be struggling, and can be useful in stimulating dialogue and increased awareness regarding factors contributing to sexual boundary transgressions (CHRE 2008; Fronek *et al.* 2009; Peternelj-Taylor 1998) (see Box 10.1). In short, each team member gains from the "perspectives, strengths, empathy, constructive questioning, support, and caring" received from other team members and the team as a whole (Pope and Keith-Spiegel 2008, p.651).

BOX 10.1 CONTEMPLATING CLINICAL PRACTICE

1. For the past three months, Katherine, a forensic mental health nurse has been conducting individual therapy sessions with Mike, a client with a history of sexual offending. In their most recent session, he declared, out of the blue, 'I want to kiss you!'

- How should Katherine respond? What factors need to be taken into consideration?

2. You notice that your colleague, James, is spending more and more time with one of his female clients, a woman who has a history of sexual abuse, and who has 'fallen in love' with previous therapists. She only wants to discuss issues with James, and you have noted that he constantly comes to her defence during case conferences. Intuitively you believe that he is struggling to maintain therapeutic boundaries.

- How might you approach James about your concerns? If you were the one struggling, how would you want to be approached?

3. Over the past two months, Meghan, a seasoned forensic mental health nurse, has experienced a lot of personal family problems. Her attention to her work has suffered as a result. The nursing unit manager tried talking with Meghan about her work, and since then she has alienated herself from almost all of the staff on the unit, and spends all her time in client-related activities. One of the clients confides in you that Meghan is having an 'affair' with one of the clients on the unit.

- What is the best way to respond to this situation? What factors need to be taken into consideration?

Clinical consultation, coaching and supervision

Seeking out consultation with a trusted colleague, a supervisor, or one's professional association regarding sexual dilemmas that arise in practice can be an invaluable growth experience, and should be part of every forensic mental health nurse's risk management program (Gutheil and Brodsky 2008; Peternelj-Taylor and Schafer 2008; Peternelj-Taylor and Yonge 2003). Because forensic nurses may be blinded by their own personal issues, consulting with trusted colleagues – those not involved with the situation – can strengthen ethical decision-making. Simply talking about issues that may lead to sexual boundary violations decreases the power that is inherent in keeping secrets, or as Simon (1999) says, "it bursts the bubble of enthrallment" (p.45).

> You know when you start looking forward to seeing a client the next day, you begin to realize what is happening. I actually spoke with someone who had been through a similar experience, which was very helpful because she really was understanding and helped me sort of figure things out. I had the impression that most people would simply say, "You can't do that! Get yourself together – what are you thinking!" But what she did for me, that helped me, was to validate what I was feeling. It helped me to acknowledge my feelings rather than just beating myself up for feeling attracted to my client.[2]

However, it is not necessarily easy to share one's feelings of sexual attraction for a particular client, or one's behaviors that demonstrate poor professional judgment. Clearly, professional embarrassment and fear of being judged negatively by one's peers can be a strong deterrent to keeping secrets and remaining silent. Furthermore, colleagues may not have the competence to deal effectively with the disclosure, and depending on the nature of the revelation, their integrity may be challenged, as they are placed in a situation whereby they have to choose between keeping a colleague's confidence and reporting unethical behavior (Peternelj-Taylor 2003). Gardner, McCutcheon and Fedoruk (2010) have concluded that such "casual corridor conversations", referred to as "supervision on the run" (p.264), are exceedingly superficial in nature and should not take the place of formalized coaching or clinical supervision.

Thorpe, Moorhouse and Antonello (2009) support the use of a clinical coaching program, a formal process of professional support whereby veteran forensic mental health nurses are paired with novices to assist them with sorting through the clinical and professional dilemmas (including sexual

---

2   Unpublished research data from the author's study entitled 'The Lived Experience of Engagement with Forensic Patients in Secure Environments.'

boundary violations) frequently encountered in forensic mental health nursing. However, given that forensic mental health nurses are all vulnerable at some point, and not only when they are new to the specialty, clinical coaching should be expanded to include seasoned nurses in addition to those who are novices. "There is nothing about being senior, being a professional or being in a profession that makes the issue of sexual feelings towards patients any easier to manage" (Thomas-Peter and Garrett 2000, p.141). The importance of recognizing when and how one might be vulnerable cannot be overemphasized.

Formal clinical supervision, however, should be seen as the gold standard in forensic mental health nursing. When clinical dilemmas and challenges are discussed within the safe realm of clinical supervision, forensic mental health nurses are able to use self-reflection and introspection to mature and develop within their professional roles (Peternelj-Taylor and Yonge 2003). Experiencing erotic feelings toward one's clients represents a normal emotional reaction. How to manage those emotions is perhaps a painstakingly difficult lesson. Merely learning about ethical decision-making regarding boundaries is not enough, as ethics cannot simply be taught in a vacuum (Sarkar 2004). The therapeutic relationship is a dynamic process influenced by the context of the relationship, the client, and the nurse. As such, discussing boundaries in isolation of the therapeutic process is antithetical. Clinical supervision provides the best safeguard for the prevention of sexual boundary violations, regardless of one's age or expertise. Clinical supervision should be a prerequisite for all forensic mental health nurses, regardless of their role within practice.

Organizational responsibilities

From an organizational standpoint, forensic mental health administrators, directors and supervisors have a significant role to play in preventing sexual boundary violations between clients and staff members. They need to be alert to staff members who may be at a vulnerable place in their lives, and they need to be particularly mindful of the red flags that can occur when staff vulnerability and prolonged client contact converge (Fischer *et al.* 2008). They also need to investigate allegations of sexual impropriety brought to their attention promptly, as well as supporting those who have reported the transgressions. Sexual boundary violations that occur in practice have an immediate impact on all the staff, who may need to discuss their own anger and personal vulnerabilities further.

The importance of checking references cannot be overemphasized, particularly when staff offenders have been known to be repeat offenders (Fisher *et al.* 2008). Staff selection procedures should consider an applicant's vulnerability to establishing unethical relationships. Asking questions during interviews not only explores a candidate's attitudes, but also stresses the importance of boundary maintenance within forensic mental health practice (Thomas-Peter and Garrett 2000).

All staff, new and old alike, should be formally introduced to the issue of inappropriate interactions between staff and clients as part of their orientation to forensic mental health practice, as well as during ongoing professional development. A word of caution, however, regarding in-service educational sessions: while they may be appropriate for identifying or raising relevant matters, the depth of issues that need to be addressed regarding sexual boundary violations will likely not be addressed in a one hour seminar (Fronek *et al.* 2009).

CLOSING THOUGHTS

Sexual boundary violations are the most egregious form of ethical violation (Celenza 2007). Heightened awareness and understanding of the nature of sexual boundary violations within forensic settings will, regardless of one's professional discipline, contribute to effective risk management. Strategies need to be developed within forensic mental health care practice that deal with issues surrounding sexual boundary violations before, during and after they arise. Forensic mental health nurses continue to turn to other mental health disciplines to augment their understanding of sexual boundaries. Additional research and discourse on this topic within nursing is required. Research regarding the vulnerability of forensic mental health nurses in particular is warranted. Finally, advocating for ongoing continuing professional education, effective clinical supervision, and a meaningful program of clinical research specific to forensic mental health nursing is the responsibility of all.

REFERENCES

Bachmann, K. M., Bossi, J., Moggi, F., Stirenemann-Lewis, F., Sommer, R. and Brenner, H.D. (2000) 'Nurse-patient sexual contact in psychiatric hospitals.' *Archives of Sexual Behavior 29*, 4, 335–347.

Celenza, A. (2007) *Sexual Boundary Violations: Therapeutic, Supervisory, and Academic Contexts.* Lanham, MD: Jason Aronson.

College and Association of Registered Nurses of Alberta (CARNA) (2011) *Professional Boundaries for Registered Nurses: Guidelines for the Nurse-Client Relationship.* Available at www.nurses.ab.ca/Carna/index.aspx, accessed on 28 February 2012.

Council for Healthcare Regulatory Excellence (CHRE) (2008) *Learning about Sexual Boundaries between Healthcare Professionals and Patients: A Report on Education and Training.* London: Available at www.chre.org.uk/satellite/133/, accessed on 28 February 2012.

Epstein, R.S. and Simon, R.I. (1990) 'The Exploitation Index: An early indicator of boundary violations in psychotherapy.' *Bulletin of the Menninger Clinic 54*, 450–465.

Evershed, S. (2011) 'The grey areas of boundary issues when working with forensic patients who have a personality disorder.' In P. Willmot and N. Gordon (eds) *Working Positively with Personality Disorder in Secure Settings.* Chichester: Wiley-Blackwell.

Faulkner, C. and Regehr, C. (2011) 'Sexual boundary violations committed by female forensic workers.' *Journal of the American Academy of Psychiatry and the Law 39*, 2, 154–163.

Fischer, H.R., Houchen, B.J. and Ferguson-Ramos, L. (2008) 'Professional boundaries violations: Case studies from a regulatory perspective.' *Nursing Administration Quarterly 32*, 4, 317–323.

Fronek, P., Kendall, M., Ungerer, G., Malt, J., Eugarde, E. and Geraghty, T. (2009) 'Too hot to handle: Reflections on professional boundaries in practice.' *Reflective Practice 10*, 2, 161–171.

Gallop, R. (1998) 'Abuse of power in the nurse-patient relationship.' *Nursing Standard 12*, 37, 28–31.

Gardner, A., McCutcheon, H. and Fedoruk, M. (2010) 'Superficial supervision: Are we placing clinicians and clients at risk?' *Contemporary Nurse 34*, 2, 258–266.

Gutheil, T. G. and Brodsky, A. (2008) *Preventing Boundary Violations in Clinical Practice.* New York: The Guilford Press.

Love, C. C. and Heber, S. A. (2002) 'Staff-patient erotic boundary violations.' *On the Edge 8*, 1, 1, 12–16.

Norris, D. M., Gutheil, T.G. and Strasburger, L.H. (2003) 'This couldn't happen to me: Boundary problems and sexual misconduct in the psychotherapy relationship.' *Psychiatric Services 54*, 517–522.

Pennington, S., Gafner, G., Schlit, R. and Bechtel, B. (1993) 'Addressing ethical boundaries among nurses.' *Nursing Management 24*, 6, 36–39.

Peternelj-Taylor, C. (1998) 'Forbidden love: Sexual exploitation in the forensic milieu.' *Journal of Psychosocial Nursing and Mental Health Services 36*, 6, 17–23.

Peternelj-Taylor, C. (2002) 'Professional boundaries: A matter of therapeutic integrity.' *Journal of Psychosocial Nursing and Mental Health Services 40*, 4, 22–29.

Peternelj-Taylor, C. (2003) 'Whistle blowing and boundary violations: Exposing a colleague in the forensic milieu.' *Nursing Ethics 10*, 5, 526–537.

Peternelj-Taylor, C. and Schafer, P. (2008) 'Management of therapeutic boundaries.' In A. Kettles, P. Woods and R. Byrt (eds) *Forensic Mental Health Nursing: Capabilities, Roles and Responsibilities.* London: Quay Books.

Peternelj-Taylor, C. and Yonge, O. (2003) 'Exploring boundaries in the nurse-client relationship: Professional roles and responsibilities.' *Perspectives in Psychiatric Care 39*, 2, 55–66.

Pilette, P. C., Berck, C. B. and Achber, L. C. (1995) 'Therapeutic management of helping boundaries.' *Journal of Psychosocial Nursing and Mental Health Services 33*, 1, 40–47.

Pope, K. and Keith-Spiegel, P. (2008) 'A practical approach to boundaries in psychotherapy: Making decisions, bypassing blunders, and mending fences.' *Journal of Clinical Psychology: In Session 64*, 5, 638–652.

Sarkar, S. (2004) 'Boundary violation and sexual exploitation in psychiatry: a review.' *Advances in Psychiatric Treatment 10*, 312–320.

Schafer, P. and Peternelj-Taylor, C. (2003) 'Therapeutic relationships and boundary maintenance: The perspective of forensic patients enrolled in a treatment program for violent offenders.' *Issues in Mental Health Nursing 24*, 6/7, 605–625.

Simon, R. I. (1995) 'The natural history of therapist sexual misconduct: Identification and prevention.' *Psychiatric Annals 25*, 2, 31–47.

Simon, R. I. (1999) 'Therapist-patient sex: From boundary violations to sexual misconduct'. *Psychiatric Clinics of North America 22*, 31–47.

Storch, J. L. (2007) 'Enduring values in changing times: The CAN code of ethics.' *Canadian Nurse 103*, 4, 29–37.

Swiggart, W., Feruer, I. D., Samenow, C., Delmonico, D. L. and Spickard, W. A. (2008) 'Sexual boundary violation index: A validation study.' *Sexual Addiction and Compulsivity 15*, 2, 176–190.

Thomas-Peter, B. and Garrett, T. (2000) 'Preventing sexual contact between professionals and patients in forensic environments.' *Journal of Forensic Psychiatry 11*, 1, 135–150.

Thorpe, G., Moorhouse, P. and Antonello, C. (2009) 'Clinical coaching in forensic psychiatry: An innovative program to recruit and retain nurses.' *Journal of Psychosocial Nursing and Mental Health Services 47*, 5, 43–47.

Twemlow, S. W. and Gabbard, G. O. (1989) 'The lovesick therapist.' In G.O. Gabbard (ed.) *Sexual exploitation in professional relationships*. Washington, DC: American Psychiatric Press.

Chapter 11

BOUNDARIES AND BOUNDARY VIOLATIONS IN THE NURSE–PATIENT RELATIONSHIP WITH PEOPLE DIAGNOSED WITH PERSONALITY DISORDERS IN DSPD AND WEMSS: SOME FINDINGS FROM A MIXED METHODS RESEARCH STUDY

Anne Aiyegbusi[1]

Overview

This chapter is informed by findings from a mixed methods research study which aimed to establish the experiences of the nurse–patient relationship with people diagnosed with personality disorders from the perspectives of those with lived experience, that is, nurses working with people diagnosed with personality disorders and patients with the diagnosis. A sequential mixed methods design was employed, incorporating quantitative Delphi study data with qualitative insights based in the tradition of phenomenology, and underpinned by a psychoanalytic paradigm. The chapter reports on the sub-theme of boundaries. The services focused upon are a Dangerous and Severe Personality Disorder (DSPD) service for men in a high security psychiatric hospital and a Women's Enhanced Medium Secure Service (WEMSS).

1 I am grateful to WLMHT for sponsoring my project. I owe thanks to my research supervisors Professor Daniel Kelly, Janet Holmshaw and Vicky Franks. Also, I would like to thank Gillian Kelly for co-facilitating the service user focus groups.

INTRODUCTION

The nurse–patient relationship

The nurse–patient relationship may best be described as a one-to-one professional relationship characterised by a phased interpersonal process between nurse and patient which is promulgated through the nurse's use of self during interactions and communications, organised within an appropriate theoretical framework. Evans (2007) explains that for the nurse–patient relationship to be therapeutic, there has to be an attachment effect whereby the patient feels sufficiently 'held' within the relationship to contemplate and engage in interpersonal change. Attachment is created via the unconscious process of transference, or in other words, the patient's emotional reaction to the nurse (based upon their experiences with earlier attachment figures, usually parents) within the therapeutic engagement that occurs between nurse and patient. The aim is to help the patient recover from a position of distress and dependency towards increasing self-care, independence and wellness (Altschul 1972; Gallop and O'Brien 2003; Lego 1999; Moyle 2003; Peplau 1952; Rask and Brunt 2007; Shattell *et al.* 2006).

Stockwell (1972) found that increased quality of interpersonal care provided by nurses was associated with higher rates of recovery from illness. Stockwell's findings provide an impetus for the provision of high-quality interpersonal relationships between patients and nurses. Patients have reported that when it works well, the nurse–patient relationship has a crucial role to play in supporting recovery from mental ill-health (Breeze and Repper 1998; Carrigan 1994; Coatsworthy-Puspoky, Forchuck and Ward-Griffin 2006; Forchuck 1995; Forchuck and Reynolds 2001).

Boundaries and the nurse–patient relationship

The nurse–patient relationship is widely accepted as the main therapeutic tool employed within mental health nursing. In order to utilise the relationship as a therapeutic tool to support the patient's recovery, the nurse purposefully employs his/her interpersonal engagement skills to encourage emotional closeness and in turn produce a bond between themself and the patients they work with. It is within this interpersonal context that the healing and recovery-promoting components of the relationship are believed to be activated (Evans 2007; Gardner 2010). Indeed, a secure attachment within the boundaries of the nurse–patient relationship is arguably the essence of mental health nursing practice (Holyoake 1998) and provides the foundation from where difficult work can take place (Gardner 2010). Because of both the emotional intimacy and the power differentials involved in mental health nursing care, the patient is potentially vulnerable to unprofessional behaviour such as exploitation and abuse by nurses who for one reason or another may be unable to operate within the bounds of their professional role (Gallop 1993; Peternelj-Taylor 2002; Sheets 2001). This may especially be the case for patients residing in long-term treatment settings, with those in secure environments being all the more susceptible, especially when they are perceived solely as perpetrators of abuse and trauma to the extent that recognition of their vulnerability is eclipsed (Thomas-Peter and Garrett 2000).

Professional and therapeutic boundaries which the nurse is responsible for establishing and maintaining therefore protect the patient, the nurse and the therapeutic process (Peternelj-Taylor 2002). However, the interpersonal boundaries usually referred to in the nurse–patient relationship are a 'social conceptualisation' (Gardner 2010, p.145) rather than visible or tangible signposts. As such, boundaries within interpersonal engagement have been regarded as occurring along a continuum, with under-involvement at one end and over-involvement at the other. Both under-involvement and over-involvement are regarded as crossing therapeutic boundaries with an area in the centre of the continuum representing boundaried and therefore professional practice (Peternelj-Taylor 2002; Sheets 2001).

The nurse–patient relationship with people diagnosed with personality disorders

The research literature focusing on the nurse–patient relationship with people diagnosed with personality disorders suggests that nurses in acute and forensic inpatient settings often struggle to work therapeutically with this client group (Bowers 2002; Woollaston and Hixenbaugh 2008). The available service user literature indicates that patients often feel alienated or misrepresented by their diagnoses and that they are frequently treated with prejudice and negative attitudes by mental health care professionals (Castillo 2003; Fallon 2003; Rogers and Dunne 2011). Added to this picture is the history of personality disorder services in British high security psychiatric hospitals. For example, a public inquiry (Department of Health 1999a) identified serious breaches of security and criminal activity occurring in a personality disorder unit for men in one of the hospitals. In order to engage in the severity of subversive and criminal acts, patients had been supported by some members of staff. Some of the members of staff had apparently deliberately and consciously colluded with the patients, while others had 'blindly' collaborated in the belief that they had been working within their professional roles. The capacity of some of the patients to 'condition' professionals, including senior clinicians, in the unconscious transgression of boundaries has raised particular concerns (Department of Health 1999a; Bowers 2002).

Key criteria have been identified within the literature as being important to consider in the development of mental health services for people with personality disorders; these also indicate what makes the management of therapeutic relationships with people who have these diagnoses so difficult to achieve. That is, re-enactments of the patients' prior traumatic and/or offending histories take place within current interpersonal relationships where painful feelings, that cannot yet be verbalised, are expressed through behaviours and other communications. These behaviours and communications can have a negative or distorting emotional impact on other people, especially those tasked with providing care and treatment. From the patient's perspective, these behaviours and communications may be unconscious and complex expressions, belying attempts to seek care for unfathomable, impossible to verbally articulate but nevertheless distressing emotional states (Adshead 1998; Cremin *et al.* 1995; Henderson 1974; Hinshelwood 2002; Norton 1997). Tragically, the very behaviours and communications that these patients employ in an attempt to seek help all too often leave them painfully alienated from support and care, to the extent that re-enactments of the very traumatic circumstances that left them so compromised in the first place get repeated within the health care system (Cremin *et al.* 1995; Hinshelwood 2002). Morris (2004, p.71), in describing repetitive compulsion as present in the behavioural repertoires of inmates at Grendon, a psychotherapeutic prison for men with severe personality disorders in the UK, portrays the interrelationship between trauma and offending: '…the meaning of the offending behaviour can be understood, and it can be put in the context of a cycling repetition compulsion that usually has its origins in childhood traumas.'

There appears to be a risk that professional carers who are unable to manage the intense emotional impact involved in working interpersonally with people who have personality disorders may end up unwittingly involved in re-enactments of patients' prior trauma or offending (Adshead 1998; Castillo 2003; Cremin *et al.* 1995; Davies 1996; Hinshelwood 2002; Kurtz 2005). As such, clinicians' boundary transgressions mediate the process of re-enactment. The apparently unconscious roots of these key characteristics have not yet been fully described through health care research but are often all too evident to the practising clinician. Indeed, Kurtz (2002), in identifying a gap in the forensic mental health research, explains that it is important to begin to apply methodologies that will establish the unconscious processes employed by staff attempting to manage therapeutic relationships with serious offenders. It is for those reasons that a theoretical framework derived from psychoanalysis was incorporated within this study. Psychoanalysis offers an established theoretical and practical base for explaining and suggesting how professionals might remain within their authorised roles and work therapeutically with the emotional impact of intense interpersonal phenomena, including unconscious processes associated with patients' negative developmental experiences (Cremin *et al.* 1995; Hinshelwood 2002; Winship 1995a, 1995b). It is intended for this chapter to make a contribution towards elucidating some of the complexities of interpersonal relating within forensic services for people diagnosed with personality disorders, from the perspective of boundary phenomena within the nurse–patient relationship.

BRIEF OVERVIEW OF RESEARCH SETTINGS
The following section provides a brief overview of the DSPD service and WEMSS in order to provide some points of orientation for the reader.

DSPD service
Following a number of high-profile offences committed by severely personality disordered men in England during the late 1990s, attention was focused on the potential risk that such people present to the public once released from prison. Such men had completed prison sentences but remained a risk to the public. Their severe personality disorders had not been considered treatable within the provisions of the Mental Health Act and so they had not been detained in secure mental health services. A public inquiry into a personality disorder unit for men in a high security psychiatric hospital (Department of Health 1999a) raised awareness of a cohort of patients who were detained in secure hospitals but who continued to subvert security policies, engage in serious offending within those institutions and appeared unresponsive to treatment offered. The British government's response to this picture was to propose changes to how such people who were considered to be 'dangerous and severely personality disordered' (DSPD) would be managed in the future (Department of Health 1999b). DSPD services were proposed. Admission criteria included that the person be at very high risk of causing serious harm to other people, have severe personality disorder with high psychopathy scores as measured by the revised psychopathy checklist (PCL-R: Hare 1991, 2003) and that personality disorder and risk were functionally linked.

Controversial from the start, there was considerable opposition to these services, primarily because people could be detained for an offence they might commit in the future and frequently after already completing lengthy prison sentences for previous offending. There was also opposition to the term 'dangerous and severe personality disorder' which was considered by some to be an invalid construct. Additionally, concerns were raised about the treatability of this population in health settings (Hogue *et al.* 2007). A series of pilot projects to establish whether DSPD services were viable (Department of Health, Home Office and HM Prison Service 2004) were set up. Two pilot services for men were developed in high security psychiatric hospitals and two for men and one for women in prisons. This study took place in one of the high security psychiatric hospital pilots.

WEMSS

The WEMSS was conceived through the national women's mental health strategy (Department of Health 2002, 2003). It was recognised that many women had been detained in high security psychiatric hospitals because of the complexity of their mental health problems and challenging behaviours that could not be managed within lower levels of security rather than because of their offending histories or risk to the public. As a result, a new type of gender-sensitive medium secure service was piloted on three sites within the United Kingdom. These WEMSS services set out to provide enhanced relational security and therefore match the complexity of the patients' needs with a sophisticated therapeutic programme.

METHODOLOGY

Ethical approval

Ethical approval was sought for the study and a favourable ethical opinion was received from the local research ethics committee. Permission was also obtained from the Research and Development committees of the NHS trusts included in the study.

Delphi

Goodman (1987) has described a function of the Delphi technique to be to derive expert judgements or opinion on a particular subject. Although the Delphi has attracted criticism for its apparently weak scientific rigour, there is also a body of support for its use in clarifying complex, nebulous areas of practice where only anecdotal evidence currently exists. McKenna (1994) and Parsons *et al.* (2001) have also described it as a method which can be used to gain the most reliable expert consensus about a particular issue of concern. The rationale for employing the Delphi in this study was that no current expert nursing consensus exists within a research framework that identifies key areas of clinical processes and practices for managing the nurse–patient relationship with people diagnosed with personality disorder and there is extremely limited research-based information about this subject.

A sample of eleven nurses (including some who were highly experienced and qualified senior nursing leaders) currently working in specialist forensic and non-forensic personality disorder services were asked: 'What areas of clinical nursing practice are key to managing the nurse–patient relationship with people diagnosed with personality disorders?' All participants provided written consent.

Statements received from the participants during the initial round of the Delphi were used to develop a 170-item questionnaire. The questionnaire was then sent to the participants, who were asked to rate the importance of each item in terms of relevance on an 11-point scale where 0 = unimportant and 10 = essential. This was similar to the process followed by Fiander and Burns (1998), who developed a questionnaire from the first round statements of their panel of consultant psychiatrists, which in the second round of the Delphi asked particpants to rate each statement for its importance in the care of people diagnosed with schizophrenia on a 5-point scale.

From the results of the second round, a good degree of agreement and consensus was achieved on a large number of items and so no further rounds were necessary. The items that achieved consensus were used to inform topic guides for the next stages of this study. Items which attracted final scores with an interquartile range of 2.0 or less were interpreted as indicating group consensus. This was considered proportional to the method used by Fiander and Burns (1998), where consensus was interpreted by items which attracted final scores with a semi-interquartile range of 0.5 or less on a 5-point scale. By achieving an expert nursing consensus with regard to the research question cited above, it was felt that focus and direction for subsequent enquiry was achieved and the findings of the Delphi were used to inform topic guides for subsequent qualitative methods.

Qualitative interviews
Ten Registered Nurses who were working as primary nurses in DSPD and WEMSS participated in the qualitative interviews. All participants signed a consent form. Interviews were conducted in meeting rooms within the services and were audio-recorded and later transcribed verbatim.

Focus groups
Nine patients diagnosed with personality disorders and who were currently receiving treatment in DSPD and WEMSS participated in the qualitative

focus groups. All participants' responsible clinicians approved their capacity to consent to taking part in the study. All participants signed a consent form. Focus groups were conducted in meeting rooms within the services and were audio-recorded and later transcribed verbatim. The researcher was supported in conducting the focus groups by a senior nurse with considerable experience of working with people diagnosed with personality disorders in secure settings.

Analysis of qualitative data

The interviews and focus groups were recorded using a digital audio recorder. This required approval from the security departments of the respective services. All data that could potentially identify the participants, the services, other patients or members of staff were anonymised during transcription.

The method of data analysis used was 'Framework', which was developed in the 1980s at the National Centre for Social Research (Ritchie and Spencer 1994). The name 'Framework' is taken from the 'thematic framework' which is the central component of the method. The thematic framework is employed as a means of classifying and organising data according to key themes and categories that emerge from the research (Ritchie, Spencer and O'Connor 2003).

FINDINGS

Delphi

Although many of the items of the Delphi were overlapping in terms of providing statements about interpersonal phenomena in the nurse–patient relationship, those which can be clearly identified as relating to boundary issues are presented in Table 11.1. Statements are organised under sub-headings. The median score afforded to each statement in terms of participants' judgements about its importance for managing the nurse–patient relationship on a scale of 0–10 where 0 = unimportant and 10 = essential is reported. The degree of consensus as indicated by interquartile range is also reported.

Table 11.1 Delphi statements making reference to boundaries within the nurse–patient relationship with people diagnosed with personality disorders		
Statement	Median score 0.00–10.00	Interquartile range
Knowledge and understanding		
Nurses need to know that structured and boundaried relationships are essential elements of effective interventions with people diagnosed as personality disordered	10.00	1.00
Nurses require an understanding of the importance of establishing and maintaining professional therapeutic boundaries when working with people who have personality disorders	10.00	1.00
To manage the nurse–patient relationship with people diagnosed with personality disorders, nurses need to understand theories of trauma and attachment because these are relevant to understanding some of the interpersonal experiences that may occur, such as re-enactment of prior traumatic experience, the patient becoming disturbed by the nurse's care-giving and the tendency of the patient to try to pull the nurse out of their professional role	9.00	2.00
Nurses working with people who have personality disorders need to understand that the emotions associated with being idealised or denigrated are difficult to contain and there is a risk of identifying with the patient's distress and of boundaries becoming blurred	8.00	2.00
Applying boundaries in practice		
The nurse working with people who have personality disorders takes responsibility for setting and maintaining therapeutic boundaries within the nurse–patient relationship	10.00	2.00

cont.

Statement	Median score 0.00–10.00	Interquartile range
The nurse working with people who have personality disorders sets professional boundaries and then continues to have the therapeutic relationship with the patient	10.00	2.00
The nurse working with people who have personality disorders must apply therapeutic boundaries and set limits and ensure the patient is aware of what these are	10.00	2.00
The nurse working with people who have personality disorders manages the boundaries of the nurse–patient relationship, recognising that it is a professional relationship and that it is their responsibility to hold and maintain it	10.00	2.00
The nurse working with people who have personality disorders keeps to appointment times and agrees the duration of the appointment with the patient at the outset	10.00	2.00
The nurse working with people who have personality disorders remains boundaried and offers care that is sensitive and in collaboration with the multi-disciplinary team	8.00	2.00
The nurse working with the personality disordered patient is friendly but not a friend	8.00	2.00
The therapeutic milieu		
Nurses must maintain an environment with appropriate physical boundaries and a structured routine in order to provide psychological containment for patients who have personality disorders	10.00	2.00
Nurses must maintain a boundaried environment which includes following relevant policies, procedures and individual care plans	9.00	2.00

Within mental health services for people diagnosed with personality disorders, there must be an operational policy for nurses to follow in order to provide a safe and secure structured environment where care is consistently delivered within therapeutic boundaries and limits and where nurses are consistent and reliable	9.00	2.00
Complex interpersonal relationship work		
The nurse tries to think about things with the patient in advance of their happening. For example, if the nurse is going on leave and the patient knows that they do not react too well to separations. Nurse and patient could address this problem by planning how the patient may be able to talk to someone about how they feel during the nurse's 'absence'	10.00	2.00
Self-awareness		
The nurse working with people who have personality disorders is aware of the impact their absences will have on the nurse–patient relationship	9.00	2.00
Nurses working with people who have personality disorders require an awareness of the risk of acting out on the emotional impact of working with the patient and how to prevent this from happening	9.00	2.00

Qualitative findings

As previously mentioned, Delphi findings were used to inform topic guides for qualitative interviews and focus groups. Therefore, the findings reported in this section reflect elaborations from the interviews and focus groups in response to open-ended questions and probes on the subject of boundaries within the nurse–patient relationship. The process enables complex interpersonal work involved in managing the nurse–patient relationship to be described in more depth.

Complexity and risk

In keeping with the Delphi findings presented in Table 11.1, the concept of boundaries occupied a prominent position in relation to managing the nurse–patient relationship; also, nurses routinely worked with complex and risk-related boundary phenomena during their interactions and therapeutic relationships with patients.

In the DSPD service in particular, the need to maintain boundaries appeared to be at the forefront of nurses' minds, along with their conviction that the patients would manipulatively breach any conceivable boundary if given a chance:

> It's been challenging obviously…especially in terms of boundaries and trying to be consistent because sometimes you find they can be very manipulative, sort of like testing boundaries and if one wants to have their needs met they'll try and do whatever possible so I think it's that maintaining of boundaries which I've found to be quite challenging. (RN, DSPD)

Perhaps in an attempt to manage the intangibility of interpersonal boundaries with a patient group who were conceptualised as a complex and dangerous population of severe offenders, nurses in the DSPD service appeared to seek protection, structure and measurement from policy and procedure. These apparent tangibles also appeared to be grasped in an attempt to manage inevitable anxiety associated with interpersonal transactions which were coloured by systemic expectations about nurses' vulnerability to patient manipulation and deception:

> The thing I find difficult is the prevalence of deceitful behaviour and the constant pushing of boundaries. I mean, that is the nature of their diagnosis but you sort of subconsciously feel very pressured to be dealing with that every day because you know that they are going to do it and they present themselves in so many different ways every single day that you think this policy has dealt with the problem. And then the next thing they come up with another challenge and you think, 'Well, this isn't really covered in the policy.' What do you do? (RN, DSPD)

The DSPD patients were able to view the issue of boundaries within the nurse–patient relationship from a number of perspectives, including those that made links with how they have struggled with and violated boundaries:

> You admit you broke them or whatever or you weren't used to those boundaries and so they had to be reinforced to you before you got used

to them and we've broke boundaries haven't we? In different ways? (Patient, DSPD Focus Group)

Sexualisation of the professional relationship

The four men who participated in the DSPD focus group had varying viewpoints regarding the nature of their relationships with nurses but suggested that their individual needs informed the nature of boundaries within their care:

> To be quite honest with you mate, I'm not into chatting with the staff, I'm into, I'm here to talk to them on a level and that's it but beyond that level, I don't want to know about it. Somebody else might want to go beyond that level, somebody else might want to go all the way, are you with me? And these things do happen in institutions, we all know that, right, but it's boundaries that are set and boundaries that are set to individuals. A member of staff might set different boundaries to you than to me or to (patient 3) or to (patient 4), are you with me? (Patient, DSPD Focus Group)

However, some of the men expressed their wishes for closer relationships with nurses. This was ostensibly stated as a mechanism for getting to know them as people to enhance the potency of the therapeutic relationship, but one man explained that he had had a romantic relationship with a female member of staff in the past and continued to believe that such a relationship was appropriate. Another patient was able to explain how, when he had initially been admitted to the DSPD service from prison, he had found himself believing he could have romantic relationships with female nursing staff who worked with him but that therapy had helped him understand the boundaries of the nurse–patient relationship and his sexually predatory behaviour towards nurses:

> But also talking about schemas just now, what's going on in our head? We have to ask ourselves sometimes why we're asking these questions, why we're asking 'did you go out, are you married, you know, do you live locally, you know, how long does it take you to get here on the train?' We have to ask ourselves, 'Why would we want to ask those questions?' (Patient, DSPD Focus Group)

Phenomena associated with sexualisation of the nurse–patient relationship was not confined to male patients. Women who participated in the WEMSS focus group appeared acutely aware of the boundaries of the nurse–patient relationship and of institutional anxieties associated with transgressions within the relationship. So much so that this was brought to the focus group discussion in the following way when participants were asked about their relationships with primary nurses:

> *Patient 7:* 'They're always hugging us and everything aren't they?'
>
> [Loud prolonged laughter from all participants]
>
> *Patient 8:* 'Mine gave me a kiss.'
>
> [More laughter]
>
> *Patient 7:* 'No, no, no, they're very good, they're very good on here.'
>
> [Other participants' voices – 'yeah, yeah'] (Patients, WEMSS Focus Group)

Nurses could find the practical task of maintaining boundaries in the face of attempted sexualisation of the relationship by patients draining. The following quote is from a nurse from the WEMSS describing the relentlessness of sexual advances from the patient to whom she is primary nurse:

> 'I'm your primary nurse, this is a professional relationship, I'm accountable to provide a duty of care to you, I'm not your girlfriend or your lover!' and you're constantly, constantly repeating that, it's quite repetitive and sometimes it can be quite exhausting to maintain that boundary you know, that relationship, the boundary between them having these sort of fixations about your role and what you're meant to be doing. (RN, WEMSS)

There were occasions when members of staff had engaged in sexual relationships with patients in the DSPD service, usually over a period of time before the patients concerned disclosed what was happening. Disclosure by the patients led to termination of employment following disciplinary proceedings.

From the interviews it appeared that these female members of staff had gone to great lengths to both maintain and conceal the relationships and that they may have fallen into a category of sexual-boundary-violating professionals undergoing personal crises who utilise patients to meet their needs, as has been described in the literature (e.g. Gabbard 1999). The behaviour of these members of staff was felt impossible to understand, even if their underlying susceptibility was not:

> ...each of these two women who have done it were going through horrendous...ended up in divorces, were going through that turmoil beforehand, if you know what I mean, at home and so must have felt unloved and I can understand that and all that that involves but why

that then leads to a relationship where [Patient 5] can almost claim that he had sex with [former female member of staff] on the ward when no other staff were looking, I find that unbelievable. (RN, DSPD)

It is also of note that the pattern in forensic services of female staff violating sexual boundaries with male patients diagnosed with personality disorders and who were conceptualised primarily as perpetrators of abuse is consistent with that described by Faulkner and Regehr (2011) and Thomas-Peter and Garrett (2000).

A suggested safeguard against sexual boundary violations is the creation of a culture where it is accepted that clinicians will experience strong positive feelings towards their patients as part of their work. Within such a culture, discussing these experiences would be expected without blame or stigma (Gabbard 1999; Thomas-Peter and Garrett 2000). Some nurses included in this study suggested that they might not feel able to disclose such feelings within the containing spaces such as staff support or supervision provided by their service:

> You wouldn't want to say to them 'God, I'm almost having an affair with this patient' because the next thing you know, I'm convinced you'd have a visit from [very senior professional in the service]… Obviously this is all my perception, they'll probably say differently but I'm convinced… (RN, DSPD)

The struggle to stay in role!

While there are no published testimonies from members of nursing staff who have violated sexual boundaries with patients in these settings, it may be possible to understand something of their experience from what their colleagues have observed about them, from apparent near misses and from the experience of nurses who have felt themselves to be under interpersonal pressure from their patients to operate outside of the professional role. The following quote is from a nurse in the WEMSS describing how they witnessed a female health care assistant who they believed to be on the 'slippery slope' towards violating sexual boundaries with a patient and who, when other nurses intervened, struggled to assume her authorised role and eventually left the service:

> So erm, I mean we had a classic example with that [Health Care Assistant]… I think something was picked up by [Patient 6] and she got her to start doing things for her outside her role like she brought in a needle and thread for her, she brought in over 50 DVDs for her, she

brought in books for her and that kind of thing, so you could see where that relationship was going. You could quite clearly see where it was going. I think she was very oblivious to that, erm, and when you put boundaries in place, she struggled massively with it to such an extent that she just couldn't survive. (RN, WEMSS)

The importance of self-awareness, and of being able to contain the barrage of projections that are present within interpersonal interactions with patients, were seen by some nurses as essential to maintaining boundaried practice when working with people diagnosed with personality disorders in forensic settings. Recognition of their own vulnerability to becoming drawn into abusive scenarios, which may include re-enacting patients' traumatic histories as well as the technical difficulty involved in remaining thoughtful, appeared to be of particular importance:

> You can easily get into huge trouble because if you're not able to understand what you're doing and process your own feelings you might end up being a big abuser, if you like. You know, acting as an abuser, if you're not processing your feelings properly. So, if she rejects you, you might end up rejecting her back and then you become not a carer, you become an abuser. So, I do try as much as possible to try and process my own feelings and thoughts and behaviours, but there's times when I do struggle. (RN, WEMSS)

Thinking the whole time

Whether the priority was perceived in terms of changing dysfunctional, destructive relating and/or plain safety and safeguarding, the centrality of maintaining boundaries within the nurse–patient relationship and during interpersonal interactions with personality disordered patients in WEMSS and DSPD services was clear from this study, as was the intensity and complexity of risks inherent in boundary phenomena. Nurses working with these populations need to be supported and trained to think intensely and self-reflectively for prolonged periods of time, especially as they are often under intense pressure to exit their professional roles in order to act and re-enact interpersonally painful or abusive scenarios while they are engaged with the patients:

> I think that's the whole thing…that we have to keep thinking…it's about thinking really. (RN, WEMSS)

DISCUSSION

This research has limitations, especially with regard how much the findings generalise to other settings. However, it does contribute some new descriptions and understandings of the experience of boundaries within the nurse–patient relationship with personality disordered forensic patients and highlights areas for further enquiry. The strength of the study is that otherwise rarely heard voices of nurses and patients in these settings are reported within a research framework. The findings are in keeping with what has been reported in other studies about the pattern of female staff being over-represented in sexual boundary violations with forensic patients, especially those diagnosed with personality disorders. This is in contrast to most other clinical settings, in which the most commonly reported picture is of male members of staff violating sexual boundaries with female patients. The question of vulnerability to abuse by populations who are subject to long-term detention in secure settings and who are usually conceptualised by the severity of their own abusiveness and risk to others is raised here, as it has been in previous papers. Of importance for future enquiry is how the combination of risk and vulnerability with its parallel in staff might best be framed for the purpose of informing nursing practice within the context of cultivating and maintaining the therapeutic relationship.

The findings of this study appear to indicate a need for nurses to understand fully the role of intense projections and projective identification in terms of patients being able to locate how susceptible to boundary crossings or violations individual members of staff may be. Boundary transgressions such as breaching security procedures, sharing personal property and giving gifts to a patient may be good indicators that the member of staff is on the 'slippery slope' to even more severe violations. Also of note from this study is the barrage of interpersonal pressure to operate outside of their professional role that any nurse may be subject to from patients. It might be the case that nurses who are experiencing loss, crisis or loneliness in their personal lives may be particularly likely to be identified as people who might be pulled or pushed out of their professional role to the extent of perpetrating sexual or other severe boundary violations on patients. Either way, they may be the nurses who are least able to withstand the barrage of pressure and projections. It seems important that nurses understand these interpersonal processes in the light of patients' early histories. As such, the importance is raised of nurses having a coherent, evidence-based theoretical framework for organising interpersonal relationships and interactions. It would appear to be perilous not to do so in nursing work with patients who have such complex needs and whose risk of and vulnerability to boundary violations are so tightly intertwined. Crucially, such a framework should be compatible with nursing rather than merely the crude adaptation of models developed for the purpose of practice by other clinical disciplines and which may not translate easily or, indeed, safely into the nursing role of providing multifaceted 24-hour care within the patients' social and domestic environments.

Despite pressure applied, it remains to be clarified whether patients solely intend for nurses to act out of their role. It seems important to consider that the patient may not wholly wish to be abused or to abuse again, but that in order to be helped to discontinue destructive patterns of relating they need to be supported by nursing staff as well as other clinical professionals, and a crucial part of that support involves withstanding tremendous pressure to corrupt the relationship. Acknowledgement would need to be embedded in the culture of such services that this is a central task for nursing in these complex settings and that in-depth thinking and talking about interpersonal experience would seem to be crucial for the clinical work. A first step might be to acknowledge that nurses can and should be expected to think about intense and complicated interpersonal processes as part of their day-to-day work with personality disordered offenders. The final word in this chapter is from a patient in the DSPD service:

> At the end of the day you want that person to always be professional. I don't want somebody coming in here to work and professing to be a professional for 15 minutes of the hour. I want them to be professional all the hour, are you with me?

REFERENCES

Adshead, G. (1998) 'Psychiatric Staff as Attachment Figures.' *British Journal of Psychiatry 172*, 64–69.

Altschul, A. (1972) *Patient Nurse Interaction*. Edinburgh: Churchill Livingstone.

Bowers, L. (2002) *Dangerous and Severe Personality Disorder: Response and Role of the Psychiatric Team*. London: Routledge.

Breeze, J.A. and Repper, J. (1998) 'Struggling for Control: The Care Experiences of "Difficult" Patients in Mental Health Services.' *Journal of Advanced Nursing 28*, 6, 1301–1311.

Carrigan, J.T. (1994) 'The Psychosocial Needs of Patients who have Attempted Suicide by Overdose.' *Journal of Advanced Nursing 20*, 635–642.

Castillo, H. (2003) *Personality Disorder: Temperament or Trauma?* London: Jessica Kingsley Publishers.

Coatsworthy-Puspoky, R., Forchuck, C. and Ward-Griffin, C. (2006) 'Nurse–Client Processes in Mental Health: Recipients' Perspectives.' *Journal of Psychiatric and Mental Health Nursing 13*, 347–355.

Cremin, D., Lemmer, B. and Davison, S. (1995) 'The Efficacy of a Nursing Challenge to Patients: Testing a new Intervention to Decrease Self-Harm Behaviour in Severe Personality Disorder.' *Journal of Psychiatric and Mental Health Nursing 2*, 237–246.

Davies, R. (1996) 'The Interdisciplinary Network and the Internal World of the Offender.' In C. Cordess and M. Cox (eds) *Forensic Psychotherapy: Crime, Psychodynamics and the Offender Patient*. 2 vols. London: Jessica Kingsley Publishers.

Department of Health (1999a) *Report of the Committee of Inquiry into the Personality Disorder Unit, Ashworth Special Hospital*. London: The Stationery Office.

Department of Health (1999b) *Managing Dangerous People with Severe Personality Disorders. Proposals for Policy Development*. London: Home Office.

Department of Health (2002) *Into the Mainstream: Consultation Paper about Women's Mental Health Strategy*.

Department of Health (2003) *Mainstreaming Gender: Implementing the Women's Mental Health Strategy*.

Department of Health, Home Office and Her Majesty's Prison Service (2004) *Dangerous and Severe Personality Disorder (DSPD) High Security Services. Planning and Delivery Guide*. London: Home Office.

Evans, A.M. (2007) 'Transference in the Nurse–Patient Relationship.' *Journal of Psychiatric and Mental Health Nursing 14*, 189–195.

Fallon, P. (2003) 'Travelling Through the System: The Lived Experience of People with Borderline Personality Disorder in Contact with Psychiatric Services.' *Journal of Psychiatric and Mental Health Nursing 10*, 393–400.

Faulkner, C. and Regehr, C. (2011) 'Sexual Boundary Violations Committed by Female Forensic Workers.' *Journal of the American Academy of Psychiatry and the Law 39*, 154–163.

Fiander, M. and Burns, T. (1998) 'Essential Components of Schizophrenia Care: A Delphi Approach.' *Acta Psychiatrica Scandinavica 98*, 400–405.

Forchuck, C. (1995) 'Uniqueness within the Nurse–Client Relationship.' *Archives of Psychiatric Nursing 15*, 1, 34–39.

Forchuck, C. and Reynolds, W. (2001) 'Client's Reflections on Relationships with Nurses: Comparisons from Canada and Scotland.' *Journal of Psychiatric and Mental Health Nursing 8*, 45–51.

Gabbard, G.O. (1999) 'Lessons to be Learned from the Study of Sexual Boundary Violations.' *American Journal of Psychotherapy 50*, 3, 311–322.

Gallop, R. (1993) 'Sexual Contact Between Nurses and Patients.' *Canadian Nurse 89*, 2, 28–31.

Gallop, R. and O'Brien, L. (2003) 'Re-establishing Psychodynamic Theory as Foundational Knowledge for Psychiatric/Mental Health Nursing.' *Issues in Mental Health Nursing 24*, 213–227.

Gardner, A. (2010) 'Therapeutic Friendliness and the Development of Therapeutic Leverage by Mental Health Nurses in Community Rehabilitation Settings.' *Contemporary Nurse 34*, 2, 140–148.

Goodman, C.M. (1987) 'The Delphi Technique: A Critique.' *Journal of Advanced Nursing 12*, 729–734.

Hare, R.D. (1991) *The Psychopathy Checklist – Revised*. Toronto: Multi Health Systems.

Hare, R.D. (2003) *Manual for the Revised Psychopathy Checklist*. Toronto: Multi Health Systems.

Henderson, S. (1974) 'Care-Eliciting Behaviour in Man.' *Journal of Nervous and Mental Disorder 15*, 3, 172–181.

Hinshelwood, R.D. (2002) 'Abusive Help – Helping Abuse: The Psychodynamic Impact of Severe Personality Disorder on Caring Institutions.' *Criminal Behaviour and Mental Health 12*, S20–S30.

Hogue, T.E., Jones, L., Talkes, K. and Tennant, A. (2007) 'The Peaks: A Clinical Service for those with Dangerous and Severe Personality Disorder.' *Psychology, Crime and Law 13*, 1, 57–68.

Holyoake, D. (1998) 'Disentangling Caring from Love in a Nurse–Patient Relationship.' *Nursing Times 94*, 49, 56–58.

Kurtz, A. (2002) 'A Psychoanalytic View of Two Forensic Mental Health Services.' *Criminal Behaviour and Mental Health 12*, 68–80.

Kurtz, A. (2005) 'The Needs of Staff who Care for People with a Diagnosis of Personality Disorders who are Considered a Risk to Others.' *Journal of Forensic Psychiatry and Psychology 16*, 2, 399–422.

Lego, S. (1999) 'The One-to-One Nurse Patient Relationship.' *Perspectives in Psychiatric Care 35*, 4, 4–22.

McKenna, H.P. (1994) 'The Delphi Technique: A Worthwhile Research Approach for Nursing?' *Journal of Advanced Nursing 19*, 1221–1225.

Morris, M. (2004) *Dangerous and Severe – Process, Programme and Person: Grendon's Work*. London: Jessica Kingsley Publishers.

Moyle, W. (2003) 'Nurse–Patient Relationship: A Dichotomy of Expectations.' *International Journal of Mental Health Nursing 12*, 103–109.

Norton, K. (1997) 'In the Prison of Severe Personality Disorder.' *Journal of Forensic Psychiatry and Psychology 8*, 2, 285–298.

Parsons, S., Barker, P.J. and Armstrong, A.E. (2001) 'The Teaching of Health Care Ethics to Students of Nursing in the UK: A Pilot Study.' *Nursing Ethics 8*, 1, 45–56.

Peplau, H, E. (1952) *Interpersonal Relations in Nursing*. New York: Putnam.

Peternelj-Taylor, C. (2002) 'Professional Boundaries. A Matter of Therapeutic Integrity.' *Journal of Psychosocial Nursing and Mental Health Services 40*, 4, 22–29.

Rask, M. and Brunt, D. (2007) 'Verbal and Social Interaction in the Nurse–Patient Relationship in Forensic Psychiatric Nursing Care: A Model and its Philosophical and Theoretic Foundation.' *Nursing Inquiry 14*, 2, 169–176.

Ritchie, J. and Spencer, L. (1994) 'Qualitative Data Analysis for Applied Policy Research.' In A. Bryman and R.G. Burgess (eds) *Analysing Qualitative Data*. London: Routledge.

Ritchie, J., Spencer, L. and O'Connor, W. (2003) 'Carrying out Qualitative Analysis.' In J. Ritchie and J. Lewis (eds) *Qualitative Research Practice: A Guide for Social Science Students and Researchers*. London: Sage.

Rogers, B. and Dunne, E. (2011) '"They told me I had this Personality Disorder… All of a Sudden I was Wasting their Time": Personality Disorder and the Inpatient Experience.' *Journal of Mental Health 20*, 3, 226–233.

Shattell, M.M., McAllister, S., Hogan, B. and Thomas, S.P. (2006) 'She Took Time To Make Sure She Understood. Mental Health Patients' Experiences of Being Understood.' *Archives of Psychiatric Nursing 20*, 5, 234–241.

Sheets, V.R. (2001) 'Professional Boundaries: Staying in the Lines.' *Dimensions of Critical Care Nursing 20*, 5, 36–40.

Stockwell, F. (1972) *The Unpopular Patient*. Royal College of Nursing Research Project. Series 1, No 2. London: Royal College of Nursing.

Thomas-Peter, B. and Garrett, T. (2000) 'Preventing Sexual Contact Between Professionals and Patients in Forensic Environments.' *Journal of Forensic Psychiatry 11*, 1, 135–150.

Winship, G. (1995a) 'The Unconscious Impact of Caring for Acutely Disturbed Patients: A Perspective for Supervision.' *Journal of Psychiatric and Mental Health Nursing 2*, 227–233.

Winship, G. (1995b) 'Nursing and Psychoanalysis – Uneasy Alliances?' *Psychoanalytic Psychotherapy 9*, 3, 289–299.

Woollaston, K. and Hixenbaugh, P. (2008) '"Destructive Whirlwind": Nurses Perceptions of Patients Diagnosed with Borderline Personality Disorder.' *Journal of Psychiatric and Mental Health Nursing 15*, 703–709.

Chapter 12

BOUNDARY VIOLATIONS IN MEDIUM SECURITY

Brian Darnley, David Reiss and Gabriel Kirtchuk

Overview

This chapter explores boundary violations in the context of medium secure forensic settings, a particularly fertile setting for their enactment. The patients contained within these institutions have histories of serious offending behaviour, usually of a violent or sexual nature. By virtue of the legal requirements placed upon them they are forced into long-term therapeutic relationships with those responsible for their treatment. It is therefore not surprising that the interpersonal dynamics that have characterised these patients' lives continue to be re-enacted with staff in the treatment setting, often resulting in boundary violations which may be difficult to recognise. The authors outline an approach that facilitates greater awareness, though improving the multi-disciplinary team's understanding of the patient. If the dynamics that facilitate boundary violations can be discovered and described at an early stage, then subsequent, perhaps serious, breaches can be prevented. Caring staff are also able to begin to provide the patient with clearer insight into the interpersonal aspects of their condition, thereby promoting further psychological change.

INTRODUCTION

Why has so little been previously written about boundary violations in medium secure settings, despite this being a major issue in clinical practice? There are probably a variety of reasons but perhaps the most obvious is our own reluctance as professionals to countenance the idea that we may harm patients, or that our care can fall well below the standards we aspire to. In addition, it is also difficult for staff to think about those boundary violations that appear to originate from the patient. These are highly disturbing in that they challenge our notions of the therapeutic endeavour, in which mental health care professionals go to work to help their patients 'get better', and the idea that patients might want to corrupt, attack or even murder us for our efforts is extremely difficult to face. Instead, it is easy to see how we could be tempted to hold onto an idealised version of the therapeutic encounter: willing, compliant patients who respond to treatment by getting 'better' because of the wonderful care delivered by our 'heroic' professional staff. However, this personal and institutional defence is a denial of the sheer emotional maelstrom present on our inpatient wards. Furthermore, and perhaps even more disturbing, is that a boundary violation rarely emanates from one participant in an enactment, but is usually a complex interplay between patient and staff where both act partially conscious, or mainly unconscious, dynamics which are often a repetition of early childhood experiences. As the popular refrain goes, 'it takes two to tango'.

WHAT ARE BOUNDARY VIOLATIONS?

Observing boundaries' and 'being boundaried' are terms often discussed by mental health professionals and whilst most would profess to know what these terms mean, it is rare that much time is ever spent discussing their precise definition. The concept of 'boundary breach' tends to be used in a general and vague way, either with the concerning behaviour usually not specifically mentioned, or in a rather loose manner for inappropriate professional and/or patient conduct.

Sarkar (2004) defines the term 'boundary' in professional practice as the distinction between professional and personal identity, stating that the purpose of the concept is to keep both parties safe by ensuring that professionals and patients can be sure of their roles in clinical encounters. Miller and Maier (2002) describe boundaries as 'the limits that circumscribe the relationship between a health care professional and a patient'. These definitions emphasise the interpersonal dimension and lead us to conceptualise boundary violations in terms of a breach in the relationship between patient and professional, where roles and responsibilities occupied by each are no longer respected and one, or both, step out of role. However we should not limit the conceptualisation of boundary violations to the infringement of interpersonal boundaries. Epstein (1994) defines a boundary violation as a harmful crossing or transgression of a boundary, which is ultimately harmful to the patient and their treatment. It may be simpler to say that boundaries are violated whenever the professional or patient fails to act in the best interests of the patient. In the medium secure setting, boundary violations must also include breaching the rules and regulations.

Although the published literature concentrates on boundary violations characterised by a professional's over-involvement with a patient, in particular those that lead to a sexual relationship, far more common in our experience in medium security are boundary violations characterised by under-involvement (Peternelj-Taylor 2002). Examples of the latter are: superficial attempts to engage the patient; following staff agendas whilst ignoring patient concerns; not exploring their difficulties in any sort of meaningful depth; or physically avoiding them altogether (Friedman and Gelso 2000). Of course, this suits many patients who would rather avoid any sort of emotional contact or exploration of their difficulties. In fact, as mentioned earlier, this is usually an unwitting enactment between patient and staff which often only comes to light as patients approach their discharge. The team then starts to realise that not much work has taken place, or that a lot of work has been completed but only superficially engaged with, and there has been little real change.

BOUNDARY VIOLATIONS, CROSSINGS AND THE 'SLIPPERY SLOPE'

Gross boundary violations are usually obvious. However, smaller ones are much harder to spot and, even when detected, can elicit conflicting views from professionals, not all of whom would agree on whether a violation has occurred. In addition, the appropriateness of the behaviour might also depend on their professional discipline and seniority within the medium secure unit. Furthermore, in some circumstances a boundary violation might be considered or used in a therapeutic way and as such might be more appropriately termed a boundary crossing.

Boundary crossings are defined as deviations from commonly accepted clinical practice (Lamb and Catanzaro 1998). They are harmless, non-exploitative, and may be supportive of the therapy process. Examples might include disclosing personal information or spending more time with certain patients.

Nevertheless, this is murky territory. The problem is that depending on the nature and the extent of the disclosure, one might move from a boundary crossing into a violation – after all, therapist self-disclosure is the most common boundary violation that precedes sexual involvement with a patient (Schoener 1998). Furthermore, gross boundary violations are usually preceded by a series of less serious crossings or violations before developing into the full boundary violation. This is called the 'slippery slope' (Gutheil and Simon 2002). Boundary crossings become small boundary violations which are often justified as harmless but may gradually escalate into major breaches which are harmful to the patient (Gabbard and Lester 1995, 2003; Gutheil and Simon 2002). This may take place because of limited clinical supervision, role confusion due to broad-based demands, failure to educate oneself about their criminal history, lack of awareness of small breaches, and lack of cohesion in the treating team (Love and Heber 2002).

THE SPECIALIST NATURE OF THE MEDIUM SECURE FORENSIC ENVIRONMENT

Forensic settings are fertile ground for boundary violations. Forensic patients are incarcerated precisely because of their history of being unable to respect the social mores or boundaries of society. In medium security the overwhelming majority have mental illness. It may be difficult to distinguish between the patient's personality factors and the manifestations of their illness.

Such patients are usually admitted to the hospital unit for lengthy periods of time. Patient and professional are forced into a long-term, sometimes lifetime, relationship by the legal process. Furthermore, for patients in medium security, members of staff are working in their living environment during a period in their hospitalisation when there is usually little opportunity for any sort of leave and most patients are usually, at least initially, not well enough to engage in much therapeutic activity off the ward.

This sets up a situation in which patient and professional spend an extensive period of time in close proximity when the patient can still be substantially ill. Persecuted, elated and disinhibited mental states are common and add to what is already a potentially toxic mix. For the most part the group of patients one encounters in medium secure forensic practice are those with a long-standing distrust of professionals and authority figures often stretching back to early childhood. This situation is exacerbated by the starkness of the power differential arising from their long-term dependency and loss of liberty.

The dual function of the medium secure forensic institution further complicates this situation. Tasked with treating and caring for their patients, whilst at the same time ensuring that they remain in custody in order to protect the public from further harm, these units need to balance finely their caring and custodial roles to function effectively. Reports into failing hospitals often highlight how a major reason for their difficulties is that one aspect of their task has been prioritised over the other, leading to regimes that are 'brutal' with very little therapeutic activity, or alternatively more 'humane' and excessively permissive (Beales 2004; Tilt *et al.* 2000).

The particular characteristics of the forensic institution resonate and interact in highly complicated ways with the core characteristics of the typical medium secure hospital patient whose early history is frequently characterised by neglect, deprivation and severe abuse by a care-giver. He or she has often been placed in institutional care, where traumatic experiences were often repeated, before they start to come into contact with the penal system. Confusion then arises, in the mind of the patient, between caring and abusive experiences, which shapes their expectations of future care. They may then experience their subsequent treatment, including the dynamics of their relationships towards staff, as abusive, and may characterise the institution as being withholding, punitive and cruel, even when it is actually functioning well in providing a caring environment. It is easy to see how saying 'no' to a patient might be difficult when one is on the receiving end of such accusations.

To complicate matters further, forensic patients exhibit a deficit in reflective function and symbolic communication. They often act out what they cannot bear to feel and are unable to think about. This has already reached its climax in the index offence. The patient continues to repeat parallel enactments to that responsible for his incarceration in the treatment setting, although usually in more subtle and less dramatic ways. When the patient's life history prior to their hospitalisation is examined, it is often striking how these same key dynamics were enacted repeatedly in similar scenarios throughout their lives, usually with increasing severity, until the patient finally found concrete boundaries in the form of a prison or secure hospital which were sufficiently strong to contain their disturbance and violence. These enactments are often repetitions of central relationship dynamics from the patient's early history, which he or she has not yet processed or resolved (Kirtchuk, Reiss and Gordon 2008; Welldon and Van Velsen 1997).

Freud (1914, 1920) wrote about the tendency of patients to compulsively repeat past events and relationships in the present, especially when they could not be remembered or held in mind. He proposed that this was the psyche's attempt to manage traumatic situations, for example by reversing passively experienced relationships into ones in which there was a greater scope for active control. Freud saw the task of psychoanalysis as helping the patient to work through these repetitions within the therapeutic relationship so that what could not be remembered could eventually be held in mind, the past could be understood, and what had been lost or never experienced could be mourned.

To face these difficulties our patients would have to look at their own lives which have been full of neglect, loss, abuse, cruelty and violence. Forensic patients find themselves repeating the past as an attempt to master their histories. They unconsciously try to re-create these familiar relationships as a way of defending against the deeply seated anxiety about having to face who they are and what they have done. This form of enacting avoids the emotional processing necessary for true change.

Members of staff may find the intolerable nature of their patients' index offences and their ongoing transgressions in hospital difficult to live with. These enactments often leave staff feeling attacked, not just psychically but often physically, and temporarily disturbed in their thinking capacities. They find it hard to process the nature of the psychological tension that has been evacuated by the patient through his behaviour with such impact. In fact, team members are often so disturbed that they may also respond through action, even to the extent of unwittingly colluding with the very boundary violations they are seeking to stop. Whilst these reactions might sometimes be appropriate, they can also be a way of discharging unbearable feelings back into the patient. Alternatively, staff may feel so alarmed at how contact with these patients can feel that they retreat and avoid them, often unwittingly colluding with the commonly held patient view that they do not need any help from staff as they can look after themselves. Either scenario constitutes a boundary violation, in that both types of staff reaction ultimately harm the patient.

'IT TAKES TWO TO TANGO'

It is often interesting to observe how certain members of staff may be drawn into similar types of enactments with different patients. It seems that patients unconsciously pick out some individuals for certain role re-enactments. This is probably due to the personality structure of these particular professionals which is more likely to resonate with certain types of patient projection. When they meet the patient's projection with the corresponding behaviour that is being unconsciously sought, then they have become projectively identified with the patient's early childhood dynamics and at this point are already caught up in repeating the story of the patient's life.

So how can staff recognise and identify these enactments? In West London Mental Health NHS Trust we have adopted a variety of approaches to try to pre-empt, understand and reflect upon boundary violations within our medium secure forensic service. We advocate a combination of interventions, targeting both staff and patients. The reason for this is that for large parts of their admissions patients have limited ability to reflect on their predicaments and it is staff members who have to be helped to manage and understand their difficulties until the patients reach a point when they can take a greater part in the process.

Unfortunately, the forensic patient's capacity for engagement in this type of reflective activity, even allowing for modifications in technique, is for the most part limited. The vast majority of forensic patients in our medium secure unit, as in similar units across the UK, suffer from enduring mental illness. Even when these disorders are well controlled, the patients continue to be subject to severely handicapping deficit states in which poverty of thought and lack of insight predominate. Unfortunately, even when psychological work starts to help them think about their predicaments and they are able to start to make some tentative links, they may relapse back into psychotic states, as they are sometimes unable to bear the psychic pain that comes with insight.

Our forensic psychotherapy department, which is a resource for the entire medium secure unit, provides, amongst other services, Reflective Practice groups and Interpersonal Dynamics (ID) meetings (Reiss and Kirtchuk 2009). The former are weekly multi-disciplinary meetings facilitated by a forensic psychotherapist in which members of the team come together to think about their work and its impact on them, both as individuals and as a group. They provide an indispensable clinical forum for building awareness of how the frightening, fragmenting effects of patients on individuals and on the team affect the coherence of staff interventions. Only such awareness can free staff sufficiently to stand back and reconsider their roles in the therapeutic tasks they have to undertake. Interpersonal dynamics could be described as a patient-centred reflected practice. Through ID, staff members are allowed to tease out the dysfunctional nature of a relationship with a patient and transform it into a functional one, with appropriate interventions being included in the care plan. If members of staff are unable to examine their own emotional responses within a safe, professional environment, they remain vulnerable to re-enactment of dysfunctional relationships with patients. These essential interventions, which support the development of a true therapeutic environment, require managerial support in order to be effectively implemented within the clinical governance framework of a medium secure unit.

THE INTERPERSONAL DYNAMICS TOOL

This tool, developed at West London Mental Health NHS trust from Axis II of the Operationalised Psychodynamic Diagnostics approach (OPD Task Force 2001, 2008), has been designed specifically for a forensic population which suffers from complex needs, including psychosis and personality disorder, who present a particular challenge to the treating team (Reiss and Kirtchuk 2009). It examines transference and counter-transference phenomena, but in a jargon-free structured way which can be appreciated and understood by all staff members.

The method examines four perspectives present in an interpersonal relationship between service user and carer, two from the patient's viewpoint and two from that of the staff. The first perspective is how the patient repeatedly experiences others, including not only staff but also important figures from their past. The second is how the patient responds, in thought and behaviour, to these experiences and perceptions of others. These two perspectives include the interpersonal narrative of the index offence. The third viewpoint is how staff members experience the patient, and the fourth is how the professionals think and behave in response. The framework is completed during a multi-disciplinary meeting in which as many staff with experience of the patient, as possible attend. To aid the team to explore their experiences and that of their patients, they are provided with a list of interpersonal items from which they can choose those that they feel most closely correspond to these experiences and behaviours. The large multi-disciplinary nature of the meeting is designed to try to capture as many views as possible and in doing so to describe different aspects of the patient's ways of relating as well as the responses of team members.

Once the four perspectives are completed, it is possible to derive a formulation that sets out how the patient's behaviour arises from their experiences and how this in turn affects the way staff see a patient and how they respond to them. It is then possible to see how often even experienced and competent members of the multi-disciplinary team may unwittingly reinforce the maladaptive behaviours of their patients by responding to them in a way that fulfils the service user's expectations and derive an appropriate management plan for change.

Clinical example

This case is fictitious but is based on cases the authors have assessed and treated over a prolonged period of time and in different institutions.

A female patient was admitted to medium security after murdering an elderly man. At the time of the offence she was suffering from a paranoid psychosis in which she believed him to be both the devil who had stolen her ovaries, as well as the ringleader of a paedophile gang which involved the freemasons, politicians and senior members of the judiciary. She was also experiencing auditory hallucinations that told her that he had been sexually abusing her daughter and commanding her to kill him in order to save the world from paedophiles. Her psychosis gradually resolved after several months of treatment with anti-psychotic medication but she remained difficult to manage on the ward, frequently self-harming and threatening to kill herself.

Her history revealed a cruel, harsh disciplinarian mother with a weak ineffectual husband. Her father sexually abused his daughter, idealised their relationship and used to call her my 'little princess'. They formed a couple and took pleasure in keeping their 'little secret from mummy'. It later transpired that mother had known about this incestuous relationship but had let it go on because it relieved her of having to have sex with her husband, something she was highly ambivalent about, having herself been abused by her own father as a child.

On the ward, the patient dressed in a sexually provocative manner. She flirted with male members of staff and asked them intrusive questions about their personal lives, particularly their relationships. She continuously asked them for 1:1 sessions, pleading with them that only they had the skills to help her, whilst ignoring other members of staff. When these members of staff responded to her requests they found that whatever had been distressing her quickly became forgotten in the sessions and that she would then try to draw them into intimate conversations about their personal lives. Female members of staff were split in their attitudes: some saw her as a victim of horrible abuse which needed their understanding and were supportive of her requests to see male staff. Others saw her as manipulative and draining, and found it a relief that she did not request to see them. All members of staff recognised that her manner of dress was inappropriate but none of them felt able to broach this with her.

There was a general feeling amongst the nursing team that she was difficult to manage, as she was often in crisis. When her female primary nurse left to go on maternity leave, she was therefore allocated an experienced male nurse who she was thought to have formed a good relationship with. Over time she gradually stopped requesting to see other team members but instead would have a session with him on every shift he was working. This was generally seen by the team to be a good sign, as she was no longer threatening to self-harm and seemed to be developing a close and trusting relationship with him. He started doing extra 'bank' shifts on the ward, saying that he needed to earn extra money as he was going through a divorce. At night they started to have their 1:1 sessions in her room so as not to have the lights on in the main part of the ward and not 'disturb' the other patients. Over time these sessions gradually grew in length. When some members of the team questioned the wisdom of doing 1:1 sessions in her room, he reacted angrily, questioning their right to intrude on his professional therapeutic relationship with his patient and demanded an apology. They were so taken aback by his anger that they did not dare challenge him again. Several months later her periods stopped and she developed 'morning sickness' but she did not tell anyone. However, a few weeks later she developed abdominal cramps and vaginal bleeding, suggesting that she was having a spontaneous miscarriage. At this point she was highly distraught and told a female member of nursing staff what was happening to her, admitting to having a sexual relationship with her primary nurse. He was immediately suspended, then dismissed. He later lost his nursing registration and was sentenced under the Sexual Offences Act (2003).

We were asked to do an ID about a year after these events. Little had changed in her presentation and she was considered to be therapeutically stuck, engaging in minimal therapeutic activities. She continued to have frequent crises, for which she still preferentially sought out male members of staff. However, her team found it difficult to get beyond these crises to get to know her better. Due to a staff shortage a recently qualified male nurse was designated her primary nurse, despite her history. He found his 1:1 sessions with her very difficult. She made him feel very uncomfortable as she commented on his looks and clothes in a highly sexually suggestive manner, and tried to ask him about his personal life. He said that he tried to avoid doing these sessions, or if he had to, tried to keep them as brief as possible. Female team members avoided her too, feeling still very angry with her over what she had done to the reputation of their colleague and to the ward as a whole. In turn, the patient felt neglected by the staff group and said that she felt she had been left to 'rot in hospital'. She told staff that they must hate her to behave in this way towards her. She continued to dress in a sexually provocative manner and this remained unaddressed. She thought that female nurses were jealous of her good looks and the attractive stares she got from male staff.

ID formulation

According to the interpersonal dynamic perspectives, the patient largely experiences others on whom she depends and under whose care she is as *attacking* her (as the father abused her and the female nurses are jealous of her), *ignoring* her and *rejecting* her (as many of the staff team do and her mother probably did). However, she also sees some members of staff as *admiring* her (the other aspect of the jealousy, and what the male nurses do – she believes that they want to have sex with her but are prevented by the rules of her profession – and her father did).

She reacts either by *treating herself as special,* as the favourite one, or by *over-relying on* others and constantly asking people to come to her. She also at the same time is *cutting off contact* with some staff members who she feels hate her and who, as a consequence, she is unable to trust, thereby asserting herself as *self-sufficiently independent.*

Members of staff see her as *manipulating* and *attacking* as well as *behaving as though she knows best*. At the same time they see her as *cutting off contact*. They perceive themselves as either *attending and caring for her in every way* and find themselves *treating her as special* (the primary nurse who had sex with her, and some of the male staff who still liked her) or they feel *accusing* and *rejecting*, either feeling hostile to her or believing that she is capable of looking after herself and does not need them. By doing this they effectively ignore her real needs, which are those of someone who has a mental illness and who as a child had her needs ignored, was abused and was abandoned to her fate. Unfortunately, many staff end up actually either abusing her, such as the primary nurse, or by rejecting and abandoning her.

The institution contributes to the risk by allocating another male nurse to be her primary nurse. This is either an attack on her, an overestimation of her capacities, or an avoidance of dealing with her needs. In any case the nursing team had not initially seen her behaviour by having the affair as an attack on all of them as nurses. This puts her yet again in a position where she has a vulnerable man close to her who she is able to 'attack', a repetition of the index offence. She has already destroyed the professionalism of one nurse and now the institution gives her another male nurse, whilst not addressing her real needs.

Although it took a while for some staff members to see her pseudo-mature sexually provocative manner (they were again overestimating her level of functioning), the care plan which was developed included a detailed review of her mental state in order to see whether her sexually provocative manner and disinhibition was due to undertreated mental illness. It also included the decision not to avoid her because they found her difficult to manage but to deal appropriately with her dress habits as they would for any other patient. It was also decided not to give her another male nurse or therapist, as this would expose her to further risk of inappropriate intercourse.

CAN BOUNDARY VIOLATIONS BE USED THERAPEUTICALLY?

Whilst boundary violations are regrettable, it is unlikely that they can ever be entirely avoided. Furthermore, it can be argued that they provide a golden opportunity for patient and staff to help the patient understand and work through these mutual enactments. If these can be understood, they convey a huge amount of information about the patient's predicament. Understanding the part played by staff in these scenarios can be a useful way of beginning to understand the patient's particular constellation of relationship templates derived from their early experiences, sometimes even before a proper background history has been obtained. Furthermore, by developing a framework for conceptualising the ways in which patients may provoke, elicit or trigger maladaptive responses and so repeat problematic relationship patterns from the past, staff enhance their capacity to respond to future acting out behaviour with more appropriate and nuanced interventions. In the end, boundary violations are a way of engaging the patient in real rehabilitation and instead of being thought of as a rupture in treatment, they should be conceptualised as providing an opportunity for healing and repair.

REFERENCES

Beales, D. (2004) 'Pendulum Management in Secure Services.' *British Journal of Psychiatry 184*, 270–271.

Epstein, R. (1994) *Keeping Boundaries: Maintaining Safety and Integrity in the Psychotherapeutic Process*. Washington, DC: American Psychiatric Press.

Freud, S. (1914) 'Remembering, Repeating and Working Through.' In J. Strachey (ed.) *The Standard Edition of the Complete Psychological Works of Sigmund Freud, Vol. 12*. London: Hogarth Press.

Freud, S. (1920) 'Beyond the Pleasure Principle.' In J. Strachey (ed.) *The Standard Edition of the Complete Psychological Works of Sigmund Freud, Vol 12*. London: Hogarth Press.

Friedman, S.M. and Gelso, C.J. (2000) 'The development of the inventory of countertransference behaviour.' *Journal of Clinical Psychology 56*, 9, 1221–1235.

Gabbard, G.O. and Lester, E.P. (1995 and 2003) *Boundaries and boundary violations in Psychoanalysis*. Washington DC: American Psychiatric Publishing.

Gutheil, T.G. and Simon, R.I. (2002) 'Non-sexual boundary crossings and boundary violations: The ethical dimensions.' *Psychiatric Clinics of North America 25*, 585–592.

Kirtchuk, G., Reiss, D. and Gordon, J. (2008) 'Interpersonal dynamics in the everyday practice of a forensic unit.' In J. Gordon and G. Kirtchuk (eds) *Psychic Assaults and Frightened Clinicians*. London: Karnac.

Lamb, D. and Catanzaro, S. (1998) 'Sexual and nonsexual boundary violations involving psychologists, clients, supervisees, and students: Implications for professional practice.' *Professional Psychology: Research and Practice 29*, 5, 498–503.

Love, C.C. and Heber, S.A. (2002) 'Staff–patient erotic boundary violations.' *On the Edge: The Official Newsletter of the International Association of Forensic Nurses 8*, 1, 12–16.

Miller, R.D. and Maier, G.J. (2002) 'Nonsexual Boundary Violations: Sauce for the Gander.' *Journal of Psychiatry and Law 30*, 3, 309–329.

OPD Task Force (eds) (2001) *Operationalized psychodynamic diagnostics: Foundations and manual*. Seattle, WA: Hogrefe and Huber.

OPD Task Force (eds) (2008) *Operationalized psychodynamic diagnosis OPD-2: Manual of diagnosis and treatment planning*. Cambridge, MA: Hogrefe & Huber.

Peternelj–Taylor, C. (2002). 'Professional boundaries: A matter of therapeutic integrity.' *Journal of Psychosocial Nursing 40*, 4, 22–29.

Reiss, D. and Kirtchuk, G. (2009) 'Interpersonal dynamics and multidisciplinary teamwork.' *Advances in Psychiatric Treatment 15*, 462–469.

Sarkar, S. (2004) 'Boundary violation and sexual exploitation in psychiatry: a review.' *Advances in Psychiatric Treatment 10*, 312–20.

Schoener, G.R. (1998) 'Boundary violations in the professional relationship.' Available at www.advocateweb.org/home.php?page_id=47, accessed on 14 June 2012.

Tilt, R., Perry, B., Martin, C. *et al.* (2000) *Report of the Review of Security at the High Security Hospitals*. London: Department of Health.

Welldon, E.V. and Van Velsen, C. (1997) 'Introduction.' In E.V. Welldon and C. Van Velsen (eds) *A Practical Guide to Forensic Psychotherapy*. London: Jessica Kingsley Publishers.

Chapter 13

THERAPEUTIC BOUNDARIES IN WORKING WITH YOUNG PEOPLE IN AN NHS SECURE ADOLESCENT FORENSIC UNIT

Claire Dimond and Denise Sullivan

Overview

This chapter looks at what constitutes safe, developmentally appropriate boundaries in an adolescent forensic secure unit. For the purposes of the chapter therapeutic boundaries refer to all the boundaries that form part of the treatment of adolescents in an inpatient setting and not just an individual therapeutic dyad. We describe the legal frameworks within which we work which recognise children as deserving of special care and protection. Contexts in which boundaries have been violated by the adult professionals entrusted with their care and children abused are referred to. We then discuss the theory that informs it and our practice in managing boundaries within our overall ethos, which includes a significant focus on relationships in the Wells Unit, a secure unit for adolescent males which opened in June 2006.

LEGAL FRAMEWORK

Significant legislation which is relevant to all professionals who work with children in the UK is:

- *Human Rights Act*

- *United Nations Convention on the Rights of the Child*

  The United Nations Convention on the Rights of the Child (UNCRC) is an international human rights treaty that grants all children and young people under the age of 18 years (Article 1) a comprehensive set of rights.

- *Children Act 1989*

  The Children Act 1989 introduced comprehensive changes to legislation in England and Wales. Although the Act has been amended (most importantly by the Adoption and Children Act 2002, the Children Act 2004 and the Children and Adoption Act 2006), the original framework remains intact. The Children Act 1989 defines children as below the age of 18. We use the terms adolescents/young people interchangeably in this chapter.

- *Working Together to Safeguard Children*

  The legislation sets out how organisations and individuals should work together to safeguard and promote the welfare of children and young people in accordance with the Children Act 1989 and Children Act 2004. (Department for Children, Schools and Families 2010)

ADOLESCENTS ADMITTED TO THE WELLS UNIT

Adolescence can be defined as a period of transition from puberty to late teens or early twenties in which physical, psychological and social changes occur. The developmental tasks of adolescence include developing a sense of personal identity, adjusting to being a sexually mature adult, acquiring an ethical system, establishing adult vocational goals and achieving independence from your parents (Dogra *et al.* 2002). It is to be expected that all adolescents will challenge authority and the boundaries that adults set, take risks and may dabble with drugs and alcohol.

With a few exceptions the young people admitted to the Wells Unit have met the criteria for a diagnosis of conduct disorder prior to having developed a mental illness. Many have had experiences of abuse, loss and trauma and lived in areas of psychosocial deprivation which has impacted on their psychosocial development. Many of the young people's parents have not been able to provide them with adequate supervision and appropriate boundaries. Many of them have been excluded from school, used a lot of cannabis, committed offences and previously been placed in a young offender institution. Thus the young people admitted to the Wells Unit are highly likely to significantly test out the boundaries that adults set.

Adolescence does not happen in a vacuum. All young people are part of a system or systems and how they relate with other parts of the system will have an impact (Christie and Viner 2005). Normally the systems that they relate to are their family, school or work, their peers and the wider community. When working with young people in a secure setting we have to be mindful that the unit is part of the system in which they are developing and so aim to create an environment which supports them in negotiating and achieving their developmental tasks.

PURPOSE OF BOUNDARIES WHEN WORKING WITH ADOLESCENTS IN AN INPATIENT UNIT

Within an adolescent inpatient unit there is an emphasis on providing boundaries which has two distinct but overlapping therapeutic functions:

- All adolescents require their parents and/or the adults caring for them to provide clear, firm and consistent boundaries in order for them to successfully negotiate developmental tasks.

- Within any therapeutic context 'the establishment of clear boundaries is designed to create an atmosphere of safety and predictability within which the treatment can thrive' (Gutheil and Gabbard 1998). In this context a boundary can be defined as the 'edge of appropriate behaviour' (Gutheil and Gabbard 1998, p.410). Within a therapeutic relationship there is no one agreed definition of a therapeutic boundary but there is general agreement that certain parameters should be managed, such as 'time, self-disclosure, physical contact, and confidentiality' (Myers 2004, p.47).

The Department of Health's (2010) guide to relational security, which they defined as 'the knowledge and understanding staff have of a patient and of the environment and the translation of that information into appropriate responses and care' (p.5) describes clear patient boundaries as an aspect of this.

Within a secure context we need to take care that boundaries are not too restrictive. That is, that the boundaries themselves do not become barriers to treatment. Pemberton (2009), discussing relationship boundaries in children's homes, reminds us that children in professional care also need 'parenting'. Bridges (1999) states that 'a reductionist, rule-bound approach to therapeutic boundaries is not useful' (p.299). Our response to boundary challenging needs to be developmentally appropriate and therapeutic and not pathologising or over-punitive.

Boundaries can be challenged and broken both by young people and by professionals. Gutheil and Gabbard (1998) suggest that boundary transgressions by professionals fall into two categories: boundary crossings and boundary violations. Boundary crossings are benign ways in which a therapist responds to a patient. For example, a member of staff getting annoyed with a young person. They may be fully conscious of the boundary crossing, or not, and it may be appropriate. Boundary crossings may actually benefit the relationship but the main point is that they do no lasting harm. On the other hand, there are many examples of boundary violations where people caring for children in a professional context have done significant, lasting harm to the young people they care for, and these are discussed here.

WHEN BOUNDARIES ARE VIOLATED

What can we learn?

Since the early 1990s there has been widespread recognition that many children have been abused in residential homes, particularly between the mid-1960s and mid-1980s, the abuse being perpetrated by the professionals whom the state had entrusted with the role of caring for these children and young people who were both vulnerable and traumatised and presenting with challenging behaviour. All types of abuse – emotional, physical, sexual and neglect – often occurred together. Bennetto (2001) reported that there were 67 ongoing or recently completed police investigations involving 2000 former residents of children's homes, more than 400 homes or schools, and 415 suspects, and that there had been at least 51 convictions.

Levy (1996) wrote that 'the Staffordshire inquiry in 1990 put a search light for the first time on children's homes'. Total 'Pindown' (Levy and Kahan 1991) was made up of persistent isolation, removal of ordinary clothing and the enforced wearing of shorts or night clothes, a persistent loss of all privileges, requiring permission to go to the toilet, no visits, writing or reading materials, radio or television, and being barred from attendance at school. The purported 'philosophy' was to give children intense, individual attention. There was no attempt at concealment by those who promoted or enacted this so-called 'Pindown' system of control, which was in effect sanctioned by those in authority.

The Leicestershire Inquiry (Kirkwood 1993) investigated Frank Beck, who was the head of three children's homes in Leicestershire and was convicted of sexual assaults and received five life sentences in 1991. In his homes there were documented treatment programmes known as 'regression therapy' which involved treating young people as though they were aged under five years, for example dressing and bathing the child, spoon feeding or using baby bottles, the provocation of temper tantrums and restraining young people in wooden playpens and placing them in nappies, the rationale being that they would 'regress' the children so that they could be taken back to an earlier period in their life when their 'basic fault' in character had been caused so that the young person could rebuild their personality. The children who spoke up at the time both to police and to senior managers either were seen as trouble-makers who were telling 'tall stories' or were thought to be fantasising. 'Regression therapy' received widespread support, articles were published in the professional journals and a television documentary was shown. One of Beck's managers regularly signed off a children's home log book containing many incidents when staff had used harsh corporal punishment.

The Waterhouse Inquiry (2000) investigated abuse which occurred in children's homes in North Wales involving at least 650 children. *Too Serious a Thing* (Carlile 2002) looked into abuse which occurred in an adolescent inpatient unit. What is striking is that similar themes and recommendations have emerged from all the inquiries which have investigated the abuse that has occurred in settings in which children are living away from home.

The most widely used international conceptualisation of institutional abuse (Stein 2006) identifies:

- Individual direct, which could include an individual grooming a young person.

- Programme, i.e. the institution's regime or treatment programme as in 'Pindown' and 'regression therapy' or over-medication.

- Organised – although he notes that it is not evident whether paedophile networks were targeting children's homes during these years, Stein prefers the term 'organised systematic abuse' which describes the abuse that occurred over time by different members of staff working within the same home or by other adults from outside the home.

- System abuse, i.e. the failure of law, policies, practices and procedures to protect children and young people. This would include young people having multiple placements and poor outcomes from residential care.

These abuses can occur together, as in the instance when 'regression therapy' was the treatment programme and Beck sexually assaulted the young people.

The Utting review (1997) concluded that the best safeguard against institutional abuse is 'an environment of overall excellence' (p.1) and that 'safeguarding residents is inseparable from the wider purposes of children's homes, homes which meet the personal, social, health and educational needs of children are much more likely to be safe places for children than those that are not' and that abuse is less likely when 'management pursues overall excellence and is vigilant in protecting children and exposing abuse' (p.2).

The Children Act (1989 and 2004) introduced changes in law, policy and practice designed to prevent abuses happening again. However, as Stein (2006) noted, senior middle managers, field and residential social workers, the courts and the police, politicians, parents and the public were all at one time or another desperate to find a solution to this problem (i.e. the care and the control of some of the most difficult young people in the care system) without looking too closely or too critically at what was on offer once a young person was removed into care. Thus Stein (2006) comments that whilst structural inequalities within society remain, 'there are still grounds for caution' (p.17). In addition, as Utting (1997) noted, 'even the best organisations are not immune to infiltration by determined abusers' (p.5).

ESTABLISHING A SAFE AND NURTURING INSTITUTION – THE WELLS MODEL

The clinical model for the Wells Unit (Dimond and Chiweda 2011) draws from systemic and developmental theory and from therapeutic community principles (Ward 2003a). It is informed by knowledge about the developmental needs of young people, evidence-based interventions and clinical experience. We aim to give the young people a good experience of being cared for. Specifically in relation to boundaries, we are informed by the theory that institutions are more likely to be abusive when they become closed. An institution must constantly be opened up and be outward looking.

There is a focus on relationships, the relationships the young people have with their families and peers and community professionals and with the staff and other young people on the unit as well as the relationships the staff have with each other. A review (SCIE 2008) identified that young people in residential care want staff who demonstrate a clear commitment to young people, are accepting and demonstrate a warm, caring attitude, listen to them and understand and respect them, are calm and consistent, take an interest in young people, get involved in activities with them and refrain from playing power games or constantly engaging in verbal battles with them.

Therapeutic alliance is a term for a 'variety of therapist–client interactional and relational factors operating in the delivery of treatment' (Green 2006, p.425) and research in CAMHS suggests that the alliance-outcome association is higher in externalising compared with internalising disorders, where alliance ratings are uniformly high. That is, young people with conduct disorders do well if there is a good therapeutic alliance (Green 2006). A number of studies support the theoretical assumption that strong therapeutic alliances with both adolescents and caregivers are key to successful family-based treatment with adolescents who abuse substances (Hogue and Liddle 2009).

The following are core aspects of our model:

- It is multi-disciplinary – this includes team meetings, multi-disciplinary team (MDT) reflective practice with an external facilitator and opportunities for team development. There is encouragement of trainee professionals having placements.

- Staff expressing different views, with discussion about what is informing their views is encouraged. Senior staff are involved and visible in the service, especially when there are particularly difficult situations to think about and manage.

- Young people's families, friends and external professional networks are very actively involved from the beginning.

- Having a comprehensive understanding of the young person's previous experiences which informs how they may relate to professionals and understand and make sense of adult behaviour.

- Having an understanding of the group of young people and potential for difficult dynamics. Staff are very vigilant to bullying and there is a response which is discussed.

- Listening to young people – the structures and culture empowers them to have a voice in decision-making both in relation to their individual care and the day-to-day running of the unit. For example, young people are involved in discussions about the rules and procedures and taking part in cooking and the organisation and delivery of the service. The young people are actively involved in the recruitment of staff. As with staff, young people expressing different views is seen as positive. We provide feedback regarding their input, for example explaining why changes can and cannot happen and what the process is for escalating concerns and disagreements.

- There is an established link with a senior professional from social services.

- Staff education and training includes relevant safeguarding training.

- There is regular individual supervision at all professional levels which provides support, monitoring and education.

- If there are concerns about a professional's boundaries which do not warrant formal intervention there is discussion amongst senior staff to share information and a plan agreed to monitor, support and educate the professional. A view from social services is sought.

Important management processes include effective investigation procedures. The framework for managing allegations against staff is set out in *Working Together* (DCSF 2010) and it should be used in respect of all cases in which it is alleged that a person who works with children has: behaved in a way that has harmed a child, or may have harmed a child; possibly committed a criminal offence against or related to a child; or behaved towards a child or children in a way that indicates s/he is unsuitable to work with children. The guidance also includes guidelines for effective inspection, an independent complaints procedure which is easily accessible, and procedures for safe staff selection and recruitment.

SETTING BOUNDARIES

There are multiple levels at which discussion and negotiation of boundaries occurs, including with management, in the MDT, and with external professionals, families and young people. For example, parents' views are sought regarding who the young person can phone and have visit them. Boundaries are set with the young people within the context of relationships and not solely enforced through behavioural consequences. We think of the whole treatment package as therapeutic and boundary-setting with negotiation as an integral aspect. We acknowledge that we must expect some age-appropriate adolescent boundary challenging. The young people we care for initially pose a risk to others, so on admission to the unit they cannot leave it and they are restricted to certain areas by staff, and there are security items to which they have limited access.

There are a number of absolute, non-negotiable boundaries whose purpose is to maintain safety on the unit for both professionals and young people. The absolute boundaries for staff when working with young people include:

- No sexual contact.
- No secrets.
- No financial exploitation.
- No social contact.
- No physical aggression.

- No unlawful disclosure of confidential information.

The absolute boundaries for the young people include:

- No physical aggression.

- No sexual contact.

- No bullying.

- No trading.

- No mobile phones.

- No cigarettes and lighters.

There are boundaries that can be negotiated either by individual staff members or by the multi-disciplinary team. One boundary that is regularly discussed is the young person's engagement with the whole treatment programme. We expect all young people to attend education and the group treatment programme. When a young person is not engaging with the treatment programme or with certain parts of it we aim to understand the meaning of the behaviour for each young person and assess the risks associated with that behaviour. Hogan, Rogers and Hemstock (2009, p.127) said that finding the reasons behind the reluctance is 'essential' for the staff and 'critical' for the young person.

An interesting boundary that was negotiated over time was smoking. We are a no-smoking unit and our stance initially was that no young person could smoke, including whilst on leave from the unit. Smoking whilst on unescorted leave is impossible to enforce and was tested by a young person who turned 18 and legally could buy cigarettes. We then agreed if you were over 18 you could smoke whilst on unescorted leave, ensuring that the young people were aware of the health consequences. We then became aware that some of the 17-year-olds were smoking on unescorted leave. There was further discussion in the team and it became apparent that the law said it was illegal to sell cigarettes to a person under 18 but not illegal for someone under 18 to smoke. We then took the decision that we could not stop young people from smoking whilst on unescorted leave, particularly when the parents allowed them to smoke, and that it was safer for them to be open with us and store the cigarettes and lighter safely with us on return from leave to avoid them hiding them in unsafe areas whilst on leave.

Another boundary that has been negotiated is the age limit on the classification of DVDs. The unit policy initially stated that only DVDs with a classification for those aged 12 and under could be viewed. The majority of the time all the young people are aged over 15 and have regularly questioned the rationale for the policy. It was agreed that once a DVD with a 15 rating (and no higher) had been approved by a staff member and discussed with the multi-disciplinary team it could be viewed. This could not happen if any young person was aged under 15.

Whenever there is a serious incident or ongoing issue on the unit, either on the same day or the day after there is a support group. Examples of incidents when a support meeting will be held include when a young person is physically restrained or secluded, any assault or property damage, the use of illicit substances on leave and the young people getting into a lot of conflict. The young people suggested the name 'support meeting'. All young people, the education staff and other members of the multi-disciplinary team attend and a member (usually not a nurse) chairs the meeting. The chair identifies the incident or issue and the meeting provides a forum for staff and young people to reflect on the impact of the incident on everyone on the unit and to consider if things can be done differently. The meeting models to young people how they could talk about and manage difficult feelings and situations differently. It helps reinforce the purpose of the boundaries. It also helps to close an incident (Ward 2003b).

We try as much as possible to ignore 'bad' behaviour and reinforce 'good' behaviour in different ways. Our aim when managing difficult behaviour is to be non-punitive and non-retaliatory. This is not always easy. We do not have any punishment or disciplinary measures in place. Obviously on occasion we have to prevent harm to other young people and staff, and young people will be restrained and possibly secluded, but we acknowledge that restraint and seclusion could potentially cause further psychological damage. In reality the rewards the young people get are from the relationships that they develop with staff. These relationships can help contain behaviour and it is not uncommon for the young people over time to become protective towards staff.

Self-disclosure

'The idea that we can keep our personhood out of the therapeutic encounter is one that leaves us unprepared for clinical reality in all of its complexity' (Perrin and Newnes 2002, p.21). In an inpatient adolescent unit when staff, particularly nursing staff, are spending a lot of time caring for young people and are in fact in some ways in a parental role, there are many incidences when staff share personal information, although they should not disclose personal information about other staff. Staff may talk about where they have been on holiday, especially if the young person has some connection to the country, or may discuss with a young person who is leaving home their experience of becoming independent at a young age.

Gutheil and Gabbard (1998) said the question should not be about whether staff self-disclose or not but what information is self-disclosed and what the impact is on the patient. Roberts (2005) considers 'the dangers and possibilities of transparency' and offers a guide of questions to ask oneself when disclosing personal information to clients within a family therapy setting that in our view has relevance to our setting. It is highlighted that you must keep thinking about your intent whenever you disclose.

Touching

'Touch is, obviously, good medicine' according to Zur (2007, p.72) and he bases his argument on the fact that touch has been shown to increase neurotransmitters in the brain, which can have a positive effect on someone's mood as well as decreasing the level of stress factors. He also argues that 'touch can be seen as a significant factor in promoting the alliance and thus the efficacy of the therapy' (Zur 2007, p.84). An issue which can be contentious in psychiatric units is that of rules around touching. We have taken the view that a no-touch policy between the young people and staff and between the young people would be unworkable, would not meet their developmental and emotional needs and would not be therapeutic. However, sexual touching is not allowed. We also advise staff that they should not have physical contact if on their own with the young people in their bedrooms or other isolated areas. Staff will have different views about what physical contact they feel comfortable with; for example, some will put their arms around a young person, while others would not. This will depend on a number of factors including their gender, age and profession. In our view this reflects normal life and thus we have conversations with the young people both individually and within support meetings highlighting that they need to be sensitive to and respect an individual's boundaries around touching.

CONCLUSION

Within a health context, effective clinical governance, leadership and management is necessary to ensure that a culture develops in which boundary issues can be regularly discussed and negotiated. Within a secure mental health setting for adolescents, boundaries must maintain safety with humanity. Frequent and transparent discussion at a management and clinical level, including among staff and between staff and young people and their families, about maintaining and negotiating safe and developmentally appropriate boundaries is essential in maintaining engagement and in preventing boundaries from becoming developmentally inappropriate.

REFERENCES

Bennetto, J. (2001) 'Beck's appalling crimes just the tip of child abuse scandal.' *The Independent*, 8 January 2001.

Bridges, N.A. (1999) 'Psychodynamic perspectives on therapeutic boundaries: creative clinical possibilities.' *Journal of Psychotherapy Practice and Research 8*, 4, 292–300.

Carlile, (2002) 'The Review of Safeguards for Children and Young People Treated and Cared for by the NHS in Wales: "Too Serious a Thing".' Welsh Government. Available at www.wales.gov.uk/topics/health/publications/health/reports, accessed on 29 February 2012.

Christie, D. and Viner, R. (2005) 'ABC of adolescence: adolescent development.' *British Medical Journal 330*, 301–304.

Department for Children, Schools and Families (DCSF) (2010) *Working Together to Safeguard Children*. Department for Children, Schools and Families.

Department of Health (2010) *Your guide to relational security: See, Think, Act*. Department of Health Secure Services Policy Team. Crown Copyright.

Dimond, C. and Chiweda, D. (2011) 'Developing a model in a secure forensic adolescent unit.' *Journal of Forensic Psychology and Psychiatry 22*, 2, 283–305.

Dogra, N., Parkin, A., Gale, F. and Frake, C. (2002) *A multidisciplinary handbook of child and adolescent mental health for front-line professionals*. London: Jessica Kingsley Publishers.

Green, J. (2006) 'Annotation: The therapeutic alliance – a significant but neglected variable in child mental health treatment studies.' *Journal of Child Psychology and Psychiatry 47*, 5, 425–435.

Gutheil, T.G. and Gabbard, G.O. (1998) 'Misuses and misunderstandings of boundary theory in clinical and regulatory settings.' *American Journal of Psychiatry 155*, 3, 409–414.

Hogan, S., Rogers, G. and Hemstock, N. (2009) 'Inpatient CAMHS nursing: two different models of care.' In N. Dogra and S. Leighton (eds) *Nursing in child and adolescent mental health*. Maidenhead: Open University Press.

Hogue, A. and Liddle, H. (2009) 'Family based treatment for adolescent substance abuse: controlled trials and new horizons in service research.' *Journal of Family Therapy 31*, 126–154.

Kirkwood, A. (1993) *The Leicestershire Inquiry 1992*. Leicester: Leicestershire County Council.

Levy, A. (1996) 'Our dereliction of duty.' *The Independent*. 22 April 1996.

Levy, A. and Kahan, B. (1991) *The Pindown Experience and the Protection of Children*. Stafford: Staffordshire County Council.

Myers, G.E. (2004) 'Addressing the effects of culture on the boundary-keeping practices of psychiatry residents educated outside of the United States.' *Academic Psychiatry 28*, 1, 47–55.

Pemberton, C. (2009) 'What are the limits to relationship building?' *Community Care*, 13 November 2009.

Perrin, A. and Newnes, C. (2002) 'Professional identity and the complexity of therapeutic relationships.' *Clinical Psychology 15*, 18–22, 124–133.

Roberts, J. (2005) 'Transparency and self-disclosure in family therapy: dangers and possibilities.' *Family Process 44*, 1, 45–63.

Social Care Institute for Excellence (SCIE) (2008) 'Working with challenging and disruptive situations in residential child care: sharing effective practise.' Available at www.scie.org.uk/publications/knowledgereviews/kr22.asp, accessed on 29 February 2012.

Stein, M. (2006) 'Missing years of abuse in children's homes.' *Child and Family Social Work 11*, 11–21.

Utting, W. (1997) *People Like Us: The Report of the Safeguards for Children Living Away from Home.* London: Department of Health.

Ward, A. (2003a) 'The core framework.' In A. Ward, K. Kasinski, J. Pooley and A. Worthington (eds) *Therapeutic communities for children and young people.* London: Jessica Kingsley Publishers.

Ward, A. (2003b) 'Using everyday life: opportunity led work.' In A. Ward, K. Kasinski, J. Pooley and A. Worthington (eds) *Therapeutic communities for children and young people.* London: Jessica Kingsley Publishers.

Waterhouse, R. (2000) *Lost in C: Report of the Tribunal of Inquiry into the abuse of children in care in the former county council areas of Gwynedd and Clwyd since 1974.* London: The Stationery Office.

Zur, O. (2007) 'Touch in therapy and the standard of care in psychotherapy and counseling: bringing clarity to illusive relationships.' *United States Association of Body Psychotherapists Journal 6*, 2, 61–93.

Chapter 14

BOUNDARY TRANSGRESSIONS AS A TOOL FOR REPARATION WITHIN THERAPEUTIC RELATIONSHIPS

Rebecca Neeld and Tom Clarke

Overview

In this chapter, we explore the behavioural sequelae of interpersonal crises arising within the context of the nurse–patient relationship and how the dynamic repair of toxic hyper-aroused negative states creates a workable containing boundary which in turn facilitates a return to thinking. Following an overview of affect regulation from a developmental perspective, we introduce the setting and the patient. Vignettes drawn from clinical practice are used to illuminate processes described. To preserve patients' and nurses' anonymity, the individual actors described are aggregate characters rather than actual persons.

INTRODUCTION

At times of crisis, when overwhelmed by feelings, many of us will have experiences of having 'self-medicated' with alcohol, cried and shouted, picked rows with an unwitting third party, had 'duvet days' or spending sprees. At such times we break our own normative rules of behaviour and revert to primitive behaviour patterns to manage our disappointment, to mourn, to numb our feelings, even to avoid thinking at all. If and when such transgressions are pointed out to us we are unlikely to respond with gratitude and may even respond with further destructive behaviour. However, if you are lucky enough to have benefited from a normal development and good enough parenting, the resulting capacity to think means you will eventually return to 'mentalizing' by drawing upon past experiences to inform the self that the end of a love affair is not literally the end of you and your world or that there may be other explanations as to why your friend did not call you. The capacity to reflect and relate the present to past experiences is constitutive of thinking and informs our rational (adaptive) behaviour. Conversely, if one remains overwhelmed by feelings, thinking is obviated and one may continue to behave in a self-destructive or otherwise maladaptive manner. For people with personality disorders, the prospect of prohibiting or even limiting maladaptive behaviours may result in more extreme and sustained forms of destructive behaviour. Anticipating this and maintaining the ability to think or facilitating the return to 'mentalizing' is a large part of the therapeutic work that constitutes recovery.

Nurses can be preoccupied with boundaries and the breaking of them, especially when working with personality disordered people. Boundary setting can be a helpful exercise but there is a tension to be carefully managed between boundary setting as part of a safety care plan and communicating a lack of faith in the patient or an attitude of 'you will fail'. The possible consequences of boundary setting, when appropriately and sensitively considered in advance, can quicken the return to a state of mentalization.

A DEVELOPMENTAL PERSPECTIVE

In infancy the care-giver contains the child's overwhelming experience. The infant is then able to return to a state of equilibrium. This to-ing and fro-ing from hyper-arousal to equilibrium with the help of another builds a sense of self that can cope with anxiety and the narcissistic injuries that life inflicts. This process of recovery from hyper-arousal builds on previous experiences and depends on an ability to utilize the comfort of others, thus maintaining – despite feelings of humiliation or shame – the attunement with another, an attachment-seeking orientation in response to the urgent question, 'To whom might I turn with this pain?' This 'practising at coping' with hyper-arousal will lead us to become the 'container-contained' (Bion 1962) of our own emotional state, including being able to recognize that at times of great distress we may need an auxiliary ego to help us to make sense of, and aid recovery from, our distress.

For people with personality disorder the container does not develop adequately. This may be due to overwhelming sustained periods of hyper-arousal caused by abuse or through misattunement with the care-giver. The contained, that is, the emotional sphere, in which the borderline personality disordered person can operate, is extremely limited. There are strict patterns of behaviour that, if varied, cause the borderline personality disordered person to experience narcissistic rage and hyper-aroused shame (Grotstein 1990).

The failure to develop the personal capacity for containment due to environmental and internal factors means that one's ability to self-soothe will be limited and likely to be self-destructive and damaging to those from whom one might have received some comfort.

To participate in the repair of the affect-regulating system with an individual requires that the helping others be sufficiently self-aware about their personal limitations in order to have the potential to be appropriately emotionally attuned to the person's needs.

THE SETTING

The hospital houses specialist services for people with personality disorder, including those whose difficulties have become obvious after they have had children. The hospital has a planned environment managed by the nurses and patients along therapeutic community lines (Hinshelwood 1999). The patients attend community meetings and group therapy sessions, and participate in twice-weekly individual psychotherapy.

The nurses are trained in psychosocial practice and the primary nurse–patient relationship has a position of significance in the treatment. The key features of the model of nursing care are (Griffiths and Leach 1998):

- *Developmental* – in that it strives towards achieving maturity, be that of an individual, family, group or system.

- *Interactionist* – in that it seeks to understand complex personal, interpersonal and inter-group dynamics or collective understanding.

- *Systemic* – in terms of its objectives and methods.

Shift-work is managed so that the nurses spend at least three days per week on the unit. The primary nurse–patient relationship is considered from a psychoanalytic perspective and is understood in terms of transference and counter-transference. The relational dynamics can be experienced as very intense and exhausting and requires the whole team to contain the emotional labour.

Within the planned setting of the therapeutic community, the patients work, rest and play with their peers and with the primary nurses. Where the patient has a history of being abused, of self-harming and an ambivalent attachment style their internal narrative will be played out in this setting. As nurses we interact with the patients at an intimate level: going into bedrooms to rouse them and/or persuade them to come out and participate when they are reluctant to do so; helping to sort out cupboards of dirty laundry; cleaning together; cooking; and looking after others together. Nurses also encourage the development of alternative ways of coping rather than, for example, relying on medication or self-harm to manage feelings of emotional distress. This withholding of immediate relief engenders an increase in the patient's already negatively aroused state and the nurse may be experienced by the patient as similar to the care giver(s) who abused them in the past (Andreasen 2001). The job of the nurse is to know this theoretically and experientially, to be able to think most of the time while being with patients in a relationship of the here-and-now and one that recognizes the reliving of past experiences (Skogstad 2001).

The objective here is not to provide a detailed account of the hospital setting but to highlight some of the key structural processes in action, and how these structures provide opportunities for change and understanding. A clinical vignette is presented next to illustrate this.

THE PATIENT

Catriona is a 45-year-old woman receiving treatment for personality disorder in a therapeutic community setting. Her relationships with others, especially treatment services, were reported to be highly conflicted. Catriona was acutely sensitive to and sought out real and imagined failings in others which she then countered with increasingly aggressive responses, including insistent complaints that could never be adequately resolved but only seemed to escalate. The treatment aim is not one of unconditional acceptance. We seek as a team to support each other to hold on to one's self and one's mind and not to join the patients in the chaotic non-thinking space, where one wants rid of the difficult patient and the staff become familiar actors in re-creating the patient's past.

Within a matter of hours of Catriona's admission she was demanding to see the nurse-in-charge (Sam). After five minutes of this meeting, the nurse-in-charge was found sufficiently wanting to be added to Catriona's list of people to complain about.

Later the same day, Sam, the nurse-in-charge, had to tell Catriona that one of the nurses had erroneously administered 5mg Valium instead of 2mg (one could interpret this medication error as reflecting the nurse's wish to quieten Catriona down at whatever cost). Despite the nurses' initial trepidation, Catriona seemed to be impressed that they were open in telling her of this error and not attempting to 'cover it up'. However, the nurses remained wary that Catriona might use the information at a later date to berate them with. For the moment, Sam was off the list of Catriona's bad figures.

The nurse-in-charge planned a follow-up meeting with Catriona to explain that because of the drug administration error, Catriona had now received the maximum dosage of Valium she could have in 24 hours. Sam had anticipated that Catriona might understandably be very angry and upset about this and so made sure she was able to discuss alternative medication which, though it might not be to Catriona's liking, was at least available to her. By apologizing, being open about the error, outlining the implications (no more Valium for 24 hours) and presenting alternative medication options up front, Sam was able to maintain a containing boundary which facilitated thinking.

Interactions like this, where the nurse anticipates potential transgressions into non-thinking mode in order to pre-empt them, are commonplace in therapeutic communities. From a developmental perspective, considering in advance that a patient may react badly to a set of circumstances and pre-empting their reaction by meeting and talking through the anticpated distress is reminiscent of Winnicott's (1960) assertion that the mother of a new infant must actively manage the baby's environment and try to prevent or anticipate big bangs or cold draughts that could disturb the infant's equilibrium, potentially sending it into a state of disintegration.

THE FLOWERS

When Catriona first arrived at the hospital she was accompanied by an unusually large number of personal belongings which seemed to hold a great deal of meaning for her but which, initially at least, caused some anxieties amongst the staff as to the challenge of keeping and storing them all safely. Of particular importance to Catriona was her collection of orchids, which had pride of place on her bedroom windowsill. She felt that only she could look after these fragile flowers, that she derived great pleasure from doing so, and her enjoyment of their beauty helped her feel better in herself.

About a week after Catriona was admitted, the hospital received a health and safety inspection. One outcome of this was the inspector's instruction that there should be no plants in bedrooms. The instruction made little sense to staff, let alone Catriona, but there it was and Catriona had been there to hear it. There was a frightening explosion of expletives and much stomping about. Catriona phoned her friend to collect her, saying she could not stand the petty rules of the place and that 'they were always going to reject me – now they've done it!'

Catriona, like any of us, needed certain things around her to help her feel more secure. The orchids may also have expressed Catriona's paranoid and narcissistic fantasies, that with the right care (determined by her) she could bloom into a beautiful flower. However, her hope for care and transformation waxed and waned when negotiating the real world. Her perception of the arbitrariness of others' boundaries – no plants in bedrooms – fed her paranoid and narcissistic fantasies, resulting in the conclusion that 'they have devised this rule to get rid of me'. Catriona then left the hospital in despair and disgust and returned home. Over the next few days her primary nurse phoned her to encourage her to return. She was offered a meeting where she, her therapist and the primary nurse could reflect together on what had transpired.

The primary nurse also used this time to liaise with the health and safety inspectors over the issue of the plants. Given the significance of the plants for Catriona, it was agreed that her care plan would demonstrate that the plant population was being reduced. Arguably, the defining or laying down of a boundary is containing only if it makes sense to both parties. Both the patients' and staff understanding of rules/boundaries are a part of the equation. It is most likely to make sense if it fits with the patient's view of herself and her life experiences. The Trust's rule of 'no plants in bedrooms' represented to Catriona the authorities who failed to act in her interest and failed to remove her from situations of abuse, that is, authorities who were always covering their own backs.

It is of course difficult to make sense of transgressions at the time that they occur. If they can be predicted and considered at a time when there is thinking, then the recovery back to thinking is all the quicker. Care plans can be of use here to record the outputs of when thinking was possible and thus facilitate recovery. Catriona's care plan was amended to include the objective of reducing over time the number of plants in the bedroom as she became more comfortable within the environment provided for her. Her anxieties, expressed as the need to be in control and providing her own environment, would be worked with and hopefully decrease sufficiently to eventually result in a plant-free bedroom.

The meeting between Catriona, her primary nurse and her therapist was meant to determine that Catriona was sufficiently able to engage with treatment. Neither member of staff felt sure that Catriona was in a frame of mind that would enable her to engage with treatment but if she was sent home again she might never be able to return, while if she stayed there was always a chance that thinking could resume.

Catriona reluctantly agreed to the plan to reduce the number of plants in her room. She more readily agreed to apologize for the offensive nature of the language she had used to the inspector and to the community members. When Catriona was first admitted she was informed that swearing in front of children was not acceptable. If there was a risk of children hearing her ugly threatening language, she was to leave the room or would be asked to leave. Catriona had been subject to offensive and derogatory language as a child from drunken, rowing parents. This boundary made sense to her and she did not want to be in any way responsible for having a child feel the way she had when she was their age.

Finally, given Catriona's propensity to derive persecutory meanings from meetings, a written account was given to her of the meeting, noting why it was held and what the outcome was. The account was not intended to be a verbatim record but a recognition by staff and the patient that thinking might not be possible, or at least might be difficult to hold on to, and might help pre-empt getting into a non-thinking space.

SHAME

Catriona, on her return to treatment, was reminiscent of the wary Catriona from her first days at the hospital. She was anxious and insecure about relationships she had begun. She worried that the patients no longer wanted her and that staff didn't really want her back. Bretherton (1985) writes that:

> If an attachment figure frequently rejects or ridicules the child's request for comfort in stressful situations the child develops not only an internal working model of the parent as rejecting but also one of himself as unworthy of help and comfort. (p.31)

Catriona seemed to have difficulties re-establishing herself into the patient group. Another female patient had since been admitted and Catriona confided that she felt she (Catriona) now had no place in the group. Her need to be accepted created in her a feeling of humiliation. Recognition of one's needy feelings and past experience of these needs not being met, or being perceived as unacceptable, combined to create a sense of shame.

One solution to such feelings is to 'pass them on', that is, to act arrogantly and humiliate another through projective identification (Schore 2003). If a child is unable to elicit care in the usual way, for example through crying or expressions of fear, and if these attempts to get another to soothe are met with further trauma, the infant will eventually resort to an auto-regulatory strategy to modulate her potentially overwhelming levels of distress. This method of maintaining homeostatic equilibrium is imprinted into the maturing limbic system, resulting in a characterological disposition to use defensive projective identification under conditions of interpersonal stress. For Catriona to return having been sent away 'narcissistically injured', there is an 'as if' re-lived infantile experience whereby there is no one to aid the recovery of the shame associated with the injury.

Catriona managed her feelings by berating the nurse who had previously given her the wrong dose of medication and in this way was considered to be trying to 'pass on' her own feelings of shame. Although it is not suggested that this was a calculated solution, there is a sense in which it was not totally unconscious. At one point, the nurse lost her composure and suggested that it was Catriona's demanding behaviour that had led her to make the mistake. Catriona responded forcibly to this accusation, shouting at her that she is 'a PD', that 'she should get treatment' and that she is 'a useless nurse'. Catriona sought out the nurse-in-charge to complain that this nurse is 'not right in the head' and should not be working here if she is going to blame her patients for her mistakes.

A state of negative hyper-arousal was then present in both the nurse and the patient. Managing nurses' negativity and their hatred for the patient when the patient can sense it requires a cooling down period for both. The nurse has to be helped back into a thinking/feeling space where her hatred doesn't overwhelm her. The hatred is not denied – it just does not drown out everything else. The nurse has to be able to reflect sufficiently to recognize that they both had a part to play in the development of the 'shared negative state'. The nurse-in-charge subsequently organized a meeting between the nurse and patient. In the meeting the nurse apologized for losing her temper and explained that she felt worried about having made the drug error and for a short time lost her ability to think about what was going on for Catriona. The nurse went to say that Catriona had seemed 'unfazed' at the time of the drug error, while she was then the subject of an investigation. Catriona saw the nurse recover her capacity to think and to regulate her feelings. At this point, they were both involved in the process of repair. When such encounters are genuine there can be a concomitant deepening of attachment. Catriona was impressed by the nurse's openness and she went on to tell her that she could see that she is usually very good at managing.

DISCUSSION

The aim of therapy is to help people to think and to feel at the same time. When one is overwhelmed, thinking cannot happen and help may be required. One's receptivity to receiving help will be determined by past experience. This is also informed by circumstances: the nurse, subject to an investigation, had to be able to resist retreating behind a wall of 'professionalism', and acknowledge her mistake, including her failure to keep the patient in mind because of her own anxieties.

Individuals with a personality disorder can often feel overwhelmed and at a total loss to be able to self-soothe. The overwhelming feeling needs to be got rid of, cut out, buried, passed on or otherwise blotted out (Stone 1992). Drawing upon findings in psychoanalytic research, Westen *et al.* (1997) suggested that 'the attempt to regulate affect to minimize unpleasant feelings and to maximize pleasant ones is the driving force in human motivation'. A critical role of the therapist is to act as an affect regulator and to provide a growth facilitating environment for the patient's immature affect regulating structures (Schore 2003) or to complete the interrupted developmental processes (Gedo 1979). Thompson (1994) notes that affect regulation is closely connected to socialization. A therapeutic community has at its core a planned environment that facilitates the potential of affect regulation through the provision of therapy, attachment figures and socialization.

Many people with personality disorder will have endured prolonged negative states of arousal as infants or children. These intense states of negative affect are an important factor in the development of psychopathology. Their original care-givers were unable to participate successfully in the re-establishment of a state of positive affect. Opportunities for the adult modulation of affect allow for the development of self-regulation.

Within the therapeutic community it is generally a nurse who has the role of care-giver, one reason being that the nurse is more freely available than those who work in closed, time-limited sessions. For adult patients the process of 'disruption and repairs' (Beebe and Lachmann 1994, p.127) or 'interactive repair' (Tronick 1989, p.116) is played out again and again with the nursing staff. The experience of recovering from a negative affective state to a positive state with another person, who may have had some responsibility for the arousal of the negative state, is instrumental in learning from experience that negativity can be recovered from (Malatesta-Magai 1991).

CONCLUSION

For nurses in a therapeutic community setting there can be a preoccupation with boundary setting. It is as if static prescriptive boundaries and proscribed behaviours will inhibit states of hyper-arousal and the concomitant maladaptive or self-destructive attempts at affect regulation, that is, cutting, running away, overdosing. However, boundary violations undermine relationships and trustworthiness and present particular challenges for nurses when working with personality disordered patients because of the highly contingent basis of trust (Reina and Reina 2006). Conversely, in this chapter we have sought to show that it is the dynamic repair of toxic hyper-aroused negative states that creates a workable containing boundary. This can be especially powerful when the participants include those actors who contributed to the genesis of the original negative state. This requires a 'whole hospital' approach to achieve, with consideration to the organizational set-up as well as the team support of nurses engaged in therapeutic work.

REFERENCES

Andreasen, N.C. (2001) *Brave new brain.* New York: Oxford University Press.

Beebe, B. and Lachmann, F.M. (1994) 'Representations and internalizing in infancy: Three principles of salience.' *Psychoanalytic Psychology 11*, 127–165.

Bion, W.R. (1962) *Learning from experience.* London: Heinemann.

Bretherton, I. (1985) 'Attachment theory: Retrospect and prospect.' *Monographs of the Society for Research in Child Development 50*, 3–35.

Gedo, J. (1979) *Beyond interpretation.* New York: International University Press.

Griffiths, P. and Leach, G. (1998) 'Psychosocial Nursing: A Model Learnt from Experience.' In P. Griffiths, P. Ord and D. Wells (eds) *Face to Face with Distress – The Professional Use of Self in Psychosocial Care.* London: Butterworth Heinemann.

Grotstein, J.S. (1990) 'Invariants in primitive emotional disorders.' In L.B. Boyer and P.L. Giovacchini (eds) *Master clinicians on treating the regressed patient.* Northrale, NJ: Jason Aronson.

Hinshelwood, R.D. (1999) 'Psychoanalytic origins and today's work: The Cassel Heritage.' In P. Campling and R. Haigh (eds) *Therapeutic Communities Past, Present and Future.* London: Jessica Kingsley Publishers.

Malatesta-Magai, C. (1991) 'Emotional Socialization: Its role in personality and developmental psychopathology.' In D. Cicchetti and S.L. Toth (eds) *Internalizing and externalizing expressions of dysfunction: Rochester symposium on developmental psychopathology.* Hillsdale, NJ: Erlbaum.

Reina, D.S. and Reina, M.L. (2006) *Trust and Betrayal in the Workplace: Building Effective Relationships in Your Organization* (2nd edn). San Francisco: Berrett-Kohler.

Schore, A.N. (2003) *Affect Dysregulation and Disorders of the Self.* New York: W.W. Norton and Company.

Skogstad, W. (2001) 'Internal and external reality: enquiring into their interplay in an inpatient setting.' In L. Day and P. Pringle (eds) *Reflective Enquiry into Therapeutic Institutions.* London: Karnac.

Stone, M.H. (1992) 'The borderline patient diagnostic concepts and differential diagnosis.' In D. Silver and M. Rosenbluth (eds) *Handbook of borderline disorders.* Madison: CT International University Press.

Thompson, R.A. (1994) 'Emotion regulation: A theme in search of definition.' *Monographs of the Society for Research in Child Development 59*, 25–52.

Tronick, E.Z. (1989) 'Emotions and emotional communication in infants.' *American Psychologist 44*, 112–119.

Westen, D., Muderrisoglu, S., Fowler, C., Shedler, J. and Koren, D. (1997) 'Affect regulation and affective experience: Individual differences, group differences, and measurement using a Q-sort procedure.' *Journal of Consulting and Clinical Psychology 65*, 429–439.

Winnicott, D. (1960) 'The theory of the parent-infant relationship.' In *The Maturational Processes and the Facilitating Environment. Studies in the Theory of Emotional development.* The Hogarth Press and the Institute of Psycho-analysis. New York: International University Press.

Chapter 15

BOUNDARIES AND BORDERLINE PERSONALITY DISORDER

Kingsley Norton

Overview

Maintaining professional boundaries is a crucially important aspect of working as a clinician in any health care setting. Not doing so potentially jeopardises the quality of the work carried out. Worse, with patients whose formative years have been marked by boundary-breaking (via abuse and/or neglect in childhood), even the crossing of boundaries, whether or not amounting to a violation, can be damaging.

It is the responsibility of the professional to maintain appropriate boundaries, therefore, while not shrinking back from adequately fulfilling their professional role for fear of ever crossing the boundary line. Knowing the limits of one's own role and understanding the importance of professional boundaries (including when there is scope for flexibility in where to draw the line) is thus fundamental to safe and effective clinical practice.

Equally important is the professional's capacity to communicate to the patient just what is expected of her/him and to provide relevant support and education to aid in the fulfilling of their role as patient. Ideally both parties – professional and patient – know and understand what their role is and what it is not, since much successful treatment depends upon the successful enactment of their reciprocal roles.

The notion of 'boundary' can be extended to that of the role and functioning of the ward – 'what' and 'how' it aims to deliver its service. Construing a patient's treatment as a process, with a series of phases, allows attention to be paid to the phase-specific aspects, which have different task boundary implications for all concerned. In delivering their particular service to patients, staff teams can adhere to or depart from the previously discussed and agreed treatment objectives and means to achieving them.

Therefore, teams need to understand their collective role and its limits and also how to recognise relevant boundary crossings as well as violations. This requires all team members to have at least a general knowledge and understanding of one another's roles and relevant responsibilities.

This chapter addresses the above issues, including a discussion of how wards and teams might monitor their function for departures from their stated and agreed aims and objectives, specifically in relation to Borderline PD patients and their treatment.

INTRODUCTION: DEFINING BOUNDARIES IN CLINICAL PRACTICE

Doctor: 'How can I help?'

Patient (smiling): 'I want Ampicillin.'

Doctor: 'I need to know your symptoms.'

Patient (not smiling): 'I have a chest infection.'

Doctor: 'I need to know your symptoms so that I can make the diagnosis.'

Patient (rising from her chair): 'I WANT AMPICILLIN!'

Doctor (remaining seated): 'Me doctor; you patient.'

Patient (resuming her seat): 'I'm coughing up green filth…'

This interaction took place between a male ward doctor and a female inpatient, in the company of a female nurse, in the medical examination room of the forensic ward. In her mid-thirties, the patient was tall and muscular with a history of repeated imprisonment for violent crimes against male partners. She had been on the ward for one month at the time of this interaction, which had quickly become heated, with her raising her voice and rising to her feet to demand medication. The doctor had stayed seated and spoken quietly throughout. Without much time to think about how to manage the interview, he had instinctively used humour in an attempt to keep their interaction within appropriate bounds. Somewhat to his surprise, the patient became abruptly calm, providing him with his requested 'symptom' – which was in keeping with the (boundaried) role of the patient. Their short clinical transaction eventually finished satisfactorily and the patient left in apparently good spirits with her escorting nurse.

A 'boundary' can be conceived as *the line between what is acceptable and what is unacceptable for a person to do, according to their role and position*. Professional boundaries thus serve to limit the entry of potentially unacceptable personal aspects into the professionals' encounters with patients, their carers or families and also those with their own colleagues. In successfully distinguishing their professional from their personal identities, staff apply appropriate 'boundaries' and are more likely to deliver a quality service, as in the above clinical example. Applying boundaries and working within the constraints they impose therefore form essential aspects of everyday clinical practice. Often being at their most vulnerable when ill or disturbed, patients are much less able to attend to their own boundaries and so depend upon professionals for relevant protection, care and help, including support for behaving in a boundaried manner.

This definition of boundaries might seem to suggest that the professional's boundaried clinical practice is carried out at will and without effort. However, this is not usually the case. The requirement to limit the entry of adverse aspects indicates the need for professionals to strive continually to maximise positive influences in their interactions with others, while keeping negative influences at bay. In the clinical interaction reported above, it would have been easy for the doctor to have allowed himself to become drawn personally and angrily into a power struggle, thereby crossing the boundary line, to determine who was 'on top', that is, the one who should be listened to and obeyed. Managing to stay boundaried, keeping out personal aspects other than his use of humour, the doctor was able to defuse the escalating situation and complete the relevant medical task. Undoubtedly, the presence of the nurse also provided a beneficial calming influence.

The appropriate placement of the boundary line will vary, being affected by even subtle or minor changes in the personnel, roles, tasks or setting, and will benefit from discussion and negotiation between participants. However, any crossing of the boundary line is an important event and needs to be perceived as such, since a 'boundary crossing' may function as a slippery slope, leading to a harmful 'boundary violation', that is, a crossing that is damaging to the patient, professional, or both (Simon 1995). Not all boundary crossings develop into violations. In fact, crossings, in some circumstances, can serve the interests of patients. Humour on the part of the prescribing ward doctor, in the above example, might be viewed as inappropriate behaviour, hence a boundary crossing. However, although potentially a risky intervention, it proved effective in calming the patient, who then fulfilled her role as a patient in an appropriate manner. It should also be borne in mind that in keeping strictly within clear boundaries, professionals may actually fail to fulfil their role adequately, shrinking away from appropriate engagement and empathic contact with patients, their carers or families.

Within forensic clinical settings, boundary crossings and violations are particularly likely to occur, on account of the characteristics of ward environments, which include: long and/or close contact between patients and staff within the ward; patients whose early lives have been marked by abuse or neglect; and staff being required to control physically the behaviour of those for whom they are also providing care. While the placement of some boundary lines can be negotiated between staff and patients, with therapeutic benefit, many will need to be imposed by the professionals. Examples include: rules governing access to dangerous objects or equipment; the time limits of specific therapeutic activities within a ward; or clarity about who is empowered to 'order' prescription medication, such as Ampicillin. This is so as to keep the clinical setting sufficiently safe for all who inhabit or work within it, and such activity forms a part of everyday risk assessment and management.

The unstable and inconsistent nature of the Borderline patient's habitual state of mind contributes to the forensic ward being experienced as anxiety-provoking and relatively unsafe, as well as (sometimes) ineffective. In dealing with their respective stressors both staff and patients can be affected emotionally in a manner and to a degree that can be detrimental to their own boundary-keeping capacity. For staff, there are other stressors, which derive from relationships with colleagues and/or their life outside. Such factors can compromise their capacity to fulfil their role in an appropriate, conscientious and competent manner, increasing the likelihood of boundary crossings or violations or else under-performance in relation to their professional roles (Norton and McGauley 1998).

REINFORCING THE BOUNDARIES OF THE PATIENT'S ROLE

By definition, patients diagnosed as having Borderline PD exhibit five or more of the following criteria as set out in the *Diagnostic and Statistical Manual of Mental Disorders* (DSM IV: American Psychiatric Association 1994):

- Affective instability due to a marked reactivity of mood.

- Markedly and persistently unstable self-image or sense of self.

- Inappropriate, intense anger or difficulty controlling anger.

- A pattern of unstable and intense interpersonal relationships characterized by alternating between extremes of idealization and devaluation.

- Chronic feelings of emptiness.

- Frantic attempts to avoid real or imagined abandonment.

- Recurrent suicidal behaviour, gestures or threats or self-mutilating behaviour.

- Impulsivity that is potentially self-damaging (spending, sex, substance abuse, reckless driving, binge eating).

- Transient, stress-related paranoid ideation or severe dissociative symptoms.

These characteristics of Borderline PD patients thus reflect their relative inability to control core aspects of the self, such as emotions, impulses and cognitions. Such patients do not simply and deliberately elect to behave in an unboundaried manner – they often cannot exert appropriate control over themselves. As regulating their mood states is intrinsically problematic, stress from the inpatient environment (such as that deriving from a medical consultation, as with the patient demanding Ampicillin) evokes strong emotions in Borderline PD patients. Such emotions are liable to spill over into impulsive actions, which themselves represent conscious or unconscious attempts to numb or eradicate these very feelings (see above list). Depending upon the context and the nature of the 'action', such behaviour can represent boundary crossings or violations. Within the interaction concerning the prescription of Ampicillin, the boundary crossings were very minor. Importantly, intensification of the patient's emotional response and change of posture were observed early and recognised as threats to a boundaried relationship. Swift action, although unspectacular, returned interactions to a boundaried state and later to a satisfactory clinical outcome.

In order for Borderline PD patients to perform their 'patient role' adequately, they too need to know what is expected of them and therefore what is acceptable and what is not. Fulfilling professionals' expectations of them, patients would, ideally, be able to (based on Norton and McGauley 1998):

- trust and respect the professional

- articulate a 'psychological' problem

- accept appropriate responsibility for their problem

- want to be realistically rid of the problem

- disclose additional relevant (personal) information

- agree a formulation of problems and consequent treatment plan

- accept help

- comply with the rigours of treatment without behaving destructively

- maintain realistic expectations of treatment

- work to the time frame of the professional or the treatment setting

- come to terms with subsequent onward referral and/or the ending of treatment.

In practice, Borderline patients' capacities and competencies fall far short of the 'ideal'. They may not know which symptom(s) to present. Some symptoms or problems may be humiliating to reveal, for example a woman who courts sexual denigration as a way of obtaining self-punitive pain, in order to cope with inappropriate guilt feelings associated with being the victim of childhood abuse. Presenting such a sensitive 'problem', which may be her most troublesome, requires her to have a trusting attitude towards the professional, who may be a comparative or absolute stranger. Providing additional material to comply with the professional's history-taking or assessment is likely to involve her sifting through painful and embarrassing events and episodes, many of which will have been buried but not adequately emotionally processed. Such exhumation can be extremely upsetting and unsettling for her. However, having taken the risk of trusting the professional and opening up emotionally, the patient is faced with needing to close down again, at the end of the interview (or session), though without necessarily having gained any affect-regulating skills during the process. All of this potentially therapeutic process involves stress that can have the effect of overwhelming the patient's capacity to regulate emotions, impulses and behaviour, hence leading to boundary crossings, if not also violations. Sadly, it is not unusual for a patient to 'open up' in her therapy session only to 'act out' once back in her usual ward environment and routine.

Many Borderline patients will thus struggle to fulfil many of the items on the professionals' wish list and cross the boundary line in relation to others. Indeed, it may not be a psychologically healthy decision for them to reveal certain items of personal information, at least not early on in a clinical encounter or treatment episode. In some instances, those who choose to reveal such items do so from a perverse, seductive, self-destructive or placatory motive. In any case, Borderline patients find it hard to maintain a positive self-image, important for making healthy decisions about personal disclosure. Interactions with staff that require patients to examine and reflect upon their past painful events and experiences are associated with an increased risk of symptom exacerbation, which mistakenly may be viewed as clinical deterioration. Transient psychotic or dissociative episodes, with their potentially dangerous consequences, may also be precipitated by the patient's failure to cope with escalating levels of intense emotions or anxiety, which have been induced by 'therapy'.

CLARIFYING THE BOUNDARIES OF THE WARD'S FUNCTIONS

The therapeutic alliance between professionals and Borderline PD patients usually requires slow and step-wise progress via achievable clinical goals in order for it to flourish and for trust to be fostered. Setting too big a goal increases the risk of failure, which not only scuppers progress but weakens the patient's engagement in the (potentially therapeutic) process, which will then require extra care and attention on the part of the professional for its re-building. To these patients, the processing of the end of treatment or the loss of important professionals during it represents an enormous emotional and psychological challenge. This is because they have seldom been able to process emotionally the effects of prior separations and losses in their lives, being too often left to their own devices or exploited (emotionally, physically or sexually) when suffering and vulnerable, which leaves them sensitised to future 'exit' events. All the phases of treatment (building the alliance, supporting step-wise progress and termination) therefore need to be managed sensitively, not only for treatment to be successful but to prevent damage to the patient's self-esteem. Progress throughout a treatment episode is seldom smooth and continuous.

From the professionals' perspective, for positive therapeutic results to be achieved within an inpatient setting, or other setting where more than one team member or agency is involved, the following need to be embodied and collectively enacted, via negotiated and agreed protocols relating to (based on NICE clinical guideline for Borderline PD: NICE 2009):

- a shared understanding of the Borderline PD patient's difficulties, strengths, etc. (i.e. case formulation) among the treating teams/ individuals

- consistent application of a treatment plan, with information regarding any departure from this being shared among relevant professionals

- involvement of the patient, and where appropriate family, partner or friends, so that they too understand and agree the treatment aims and also the methods utilised to achieve them

- a crisis plan, so that such an untoward eventuality is anticipated and staff are not caught unprepared and so react without a concerted plan

- regular reviews of progress against previously agreed targets and timelines

- negotiating changes of key staff and transitions between teams, wards or services

- preparation of the patient for endings, transitions and discharge that occur during the treatment episode

- staff who are regularly supervised and supported via reflective practice.

From the patient's perspective, it can help to have the boundaries of their individual treatment spelled out in the form of a therapeutic contract, which if it is to be successful will need to be: negotiated with patient and carers when professionals are not unduly anxious or angry with the patient; carried out unhurriedly, with adequate time set aside for the task; and structured in order to orientate the patient about their and the professionals' complementary rights and responsibilities (Miller 1990).

Individual therapeutic contracts are undermined when patients are not provided with alternative means with which to deal with intolerable emotions. Hence their destructive or impulsive coping behaviour should not be proscribed (i.e. forbidden), unless there is a realistic, less damaging alternative provided or otherwise available to them. It must be remembered that all co-signatories to the contract, professionals as well as patients, are bound by the agreement. With this in mind, staff have a responsibility to monitor not only whether therapeutic goals have been achieved but also the manner in which this is effected, that is, whether the involvement of staff, patients, carers and any relevant others has been within the bounds of their contractual agreement.

Clearly, the ward must cater for all its patients regardless of their diagnoses and Borderline PD status and so there is always a balance to be struck between delivering an individualised, patient-centred approach and keeping the environment safe enough for all. Ideally, there is not a dramatic and extreme oscillation between custody when all therapeutic activity ceases, all privileges are rescinded and 'dangerous', everyday, objects removed on the one hand, and therapy in the form of availability of the range of multi-disciplinary input and multi-modal interventions and activities on the other. Extreme oscillations are often reminiscent of the patient's interpersonal environment in their formative years and thus they hold little or no therapeutic potential, since their usual destructive and behavioural defences are automatically erected to deal with it (Aiyegbusi and Norton 2008).

In a ward setting, for simple all-or-nothing oscillations to be avoided, the inpatient team must invest in a model of service delivery that can overarch its patients' individual treatment plans, that is, take account of the total welfare of the ward, construing it as a potentially integrated 'whole' (Badia 1989). One such model is that of the 'Therapeutic Milieu', which was developed and refined in the 1960s in the USA (Abroms 1969). This avoids a simple dichotomy of function through conceiving and providing a range of defined therapeutic functions related to a range of prevailing levels of risk. Each function is associated with defined and distinctive aims and the relevant means of achieving them: containment, support, structure, validation and involvement (Gunderson 1978). Such specialisation of function also allows the ward team to establish how closely they adhere to their own stated means for either achieving or failing to achieve their therapeutic aims (see also Aiyegbusi and Norton 2008).

MONITORING THE BOUNDARIES OF ROLE BEHAVIOUR IN FORENSIC WARDS AND COMMUNITY TEAMS

Monitoring and maintaining appropriate boundaries in Borderline PD patients within outpatient and community settings is in certain respects more problematic than doing so in a locked ward within a large institutional setting. The potential for unbounderied behaviour to go unwitnessed and/or unreported, for example, is higher and this is a source of anxiety to staff. Professionals therefore face the challenge of creating open channels of communication that convey the 'right' (boundary-related) information to the 'right' people at the 'right' time. Enabling the flow of accurate information concerning a patient's behaviour and encounters with other people such as family, friends, the public or professionals is essential for maximising the detection of boundary crossings and violations. However, achieving this is easier said than done (see Norton and Vince 2002).

In the absence of directly witnessed boundary events, 'evidence' that all is not well with a particular Borderline PD patient may sometimes need to be inferred. Thus, in addition to the overt content of what professionals (or others) report to one another, there is a need to evaluate both the manner in which the respective reports (and associated discussions) among professionals are made and also their impact (or lack of impact and response). This is to identify any departures from acceptable, that is, boundarised, practices in terms of the individuals or teams involved in treating the patient or to identify failure to engage sufficiently with the reported material (Norton and McGauley 1998). Inferences that all is not well may thus be drawn from such 'soft signs' as:

- an unusually high intensity of emotion in a meeting's discussion of a particular Borderline PD patient or particular event (perhaps arising from different staff receiving differing accounts from the same patient or from staff feeling they have 'special' expertise)

- an individual team member's high anxiety or concern, for which the professional cannot logically account (perhaps resulting from a sense that the patient has withheld important information or that their dealings with the patient have not felt authentic)

- an individual team member's expression of high anxiety and concern about a patient when nobody else shows any (perhaps resulting from dysfunctional team dynamics, which distract from or supplant appropriate concerns about the patient, or from scapegoating of the particular staff member)

- the lack of a professional's usual level of concern about a patient (perhaps reflecting unconscious denial in the face of worrying information being imparted or reflecting the presence of 'burnout' in the particular professional).

None of these inferred or soft data should be equated with actual evidence of boundary crossing or violation. However, formal inquiries into serious untoward events, often of a boundary violating nature, frequently reveal that staff had suspected or sensed that 'something was not right' in relation to a professional's or team's role behaviour. It is as if, in the absence of hard evidence, they had insufficient confidence to voice these suspicions. Staying silent, however, their passivity contributed ultimately to grossly inappropriate and damaging role behaviour resulting in major boundary violations, going unreported for months or years (see report by Council for Healthcare Regulatory Excellence 2008).

As the role performance of staff is adversely affected by high levels of anxiety and stress, all potential sources should be identified and where possible removed. Sources from which anxiety is derived include:

- uncertainty about the patient's mental state, including boundary-breaking behaviour

- staff's concern about their own physical safety

- wider considerations of safety and risk in relation to the patient's family or wider contacts within the community

- fear of criticism of their own professional judgement and competence, for example from line managers or the media.

In managing patients in the community, professionals should always ask themselves if the communication network set up around their patient is good enough. If it is not, steps should be taken to improve it, including defining the type and nature of evidence of the boundary crossings or violations that are likely in relation to the particular patient. This important information needs to be communicated to everyone in the network, with an agreed emphasis on what is priority material. Ideally, the network of professionals should be set up before treatment begins. In many cases, the reasons for this need to be spelled out and discussed with patients and, if necessary, also their family and other contacts (Norton and Vince 2002). Following the above procedure, it is likely that those involved will be able more accurately to detect from where (and where not) their current 'anxiety' is mainly derived.

Overall, the challenge to professionals working in forensic outpatient and community settings is thus to evaluate the state of health of their collective team's or network's role behaviour. This needs to be undertaken in an ongoing way and can be facilitated such as via the introduction of weekly reflective practice groups. Staff absences and irregularities, such as atypical 'sickness', unusual requests for duties/shifts or last minute changes, arguments, or sexual liaisons between any staff members, represent crossings or violations of appropriate role behaviour. All such departures from the acceptable healthy role behaviour and working practices must arouse curiosity and concern and trigger enquiry into the possibility of wider boundary crossings or violations.

CONCLUSION

Working safely within appropriate boundaries with Borderline PD patients requires professionals to be able to reflect and take stock of the current needs of their role, in relation to the overarching aims of the setting and bearing in mind the particular requirement of the patients. Ideally, within forensic health care settings, patients too know and understand, or are supported to do so, the behaviour that is acceptable, in order to play their patient role appropriately.

The professional–Borderline PD patient relationship incorporates a clear imbalance of power, making it intrinsically unstable, hence there is a need for professionals to keep in mind the difficulty their patients have with staying boundaried (i.e. fulfilling the role of patient in the context of the stresses and strains of everyday clinical transactions, such as an apparently simple request for Ampicillin). Both the in-depth psychological work and the ordinary stressors of the ward's environment inevitably create anxiety and frustrations, which can cloud judgement and impair self-control in all concerned.

The importance of the ward's interpersonal stressors on all its constituent parties (patients, staff and visitors) cannot be overstated. The physical proximity and/or emotional closeness which obtain in most forensic wards can be highly upsetting, disturbing or arousing and lead to boundary crossings or violations. Therefore, regardless of the particular situation (a throw-away comment in the corridor, a request for medication, a supportive counselling interaction, an in-depth therapy session, an entire ward-shift or complete treatment episode), the responsibility remains with the professionals to monitor and maintain the overall state of 'boundariedness' of the ward's total interpersonal environment. This is likely to require the professional at some point, regardless of their seniority, to seek support, supervision, advice from colleagues (peers, line managers or supervisors, according to the situation) or further training.

Unfortunately, boundary crossings and violations may not be witnessed or may go unreported. If they are revealed, it might be via unconsciously generated, inappropriate role behaviour within a staff team such as: unduly heated arguments; 'suspicious' (non-genuine) absences; or unhealthily close (even amorous) liaisons within the staff team. Therefore to monitor and maintain healthy team functioning (or multi-agency working, as in community settings), it is helpful to invoke the notion of a 'team boundary' related to the group's interpersonal cohesion. This can be used to test the team's capacity to deliver its collectively agreed tasks or functions and to identify aberrant or unacceptable role behaviour. This yields the potential to identify the team's equivalent of the crossings and violations of the individual professional or those of the patient diagnosed with Borderline PD.

The collective team's boundariedness is not easy to monitor. Therefore, all who work in forensic environments need to remain vigilant as to their own boundaried status (relating both to the team's therapeutic tasks and to its collective and interdependent role performance), being also aware of that of colleagues and the patients in their care. Sadly, seniority and long experience do not guarantee boundaried clinical practice. Regular, weekly 'reflective practice' meetings for all members of a team to identify and explore personal and interpersonal emotional reactions (to one another, to patients and to the work setting) are more likely to do so.

REFERENCES

Abroms, G.M. (1969) 'Defining milieu therapy.' *Archives of General Psychiatry 21*, 553–555.

Aiyegbusi, A. and Norton, K.R.W. (2008). 'Modern milieus: psychiatric inpatient treatment in the 21st Century.' In I. Norman and I. Ryrie. (eds) *The art and science of mental health nursing.* London: Open University.

American Psychiatric Association (1994) *Diagnostic and Statistical Manual of Mental Disorders,* Fourth Edition (DSM-IV). Washington, DC: American Psychiatric Association.

Badia, E.D. (1989) 'Group-as-a-whole concepts and the therapeutic milieu on the inpatient psychiatric unit.' *GROUP 13*, 3 and 4.

Council for Healthcare Regulatory Excellence (2008) *Clear sexual boundaries between healthcare professionals and patients: responsibilities of healthcare professionals.* London: Council for Healthcare Regulatory Excellence.

Gunderson, J.G. (1978) 'Defining the therapeutic processes in therapeutic milieus.' *Psychiatry 41*, 3237–3335.

Miller, L.J. (1990) 'The formal treatment contract in the inpatient management of borderline personality disorder.' *Hospital and Community Psychiatry 41*, 9, 985–987.

NICE (2009) *Borderline Personality Disorder: NICE clinical guideline 78.* London: National Institute for Health and Clinical Excellence.

Norton, K.R.W. and McGauley, G. (1998) *Counselling difficult clients.* London: Sage.

Norton, K.R.W. and Vince, J. (2002) 'Outpatient psychotherapy and mentally disordered offenders.' In A. Buchanan (ed.) *Care of the mentally disordered offender in the community.* Oxford: Oxford University Press.

Simon, R.I. (1995) 'The natural history of therapist sexual misconduct: identification and prevention.' *Psychiatric Annals 25*, 2, 90–94.

Chapter 16

BOUNDARIES AND WORKING WITH SERIOUS OFFENDERS WHO ALSO HAVE SEVERE PERSONALITY DISORDERS IN A HIGH-SECURITY SETTING

Derek Perkins

Overview

Patients with both severe personality disorder and a high risk of harm to others, who are treated over a number of years within high secure settings, are vulnerable to becoming involved in unprofessional relationships with staff. Equally, for some staff, at some times and under some circumstances, they may themselves be vulnerable to boundary crossings that can escalate into unprofessional and sometimes illegal boundary violations with patients in their care. The phenomenon is multifaceted in that it involves patient characteristics, staff characteristics, working relationships within the clinical team and the overall hospital ethos. It is also dynamic in that boundary violations tend to occur at the intersection of unfolding events for the people involved, such as positive or negative developments in a patient's pathway through the hospital, and a staff members personal life, emotional vulnerability and resilience within clinical interactions. This chapter explores these factors and provides some tentative analyses and recommendations.

PERSONALITY DISORDER

Personality disorders arise through an interaction between biological and psychosocial factors during personality development (Alwin *et al.* 2006;

Livesley 2007). Early psychosocial adversity, such as abuse and trauma, in the lives of individuals who become personality disordered result in beliefs and expectations that influence the way the self, others and the world are perceived. Typically, this includes expectations that other people are untrustworthy, unreliable, unhelpful and unpredictable (Livesley 2000).

There are two recognised classification systems for personality disorder. The International Classification of Diseases, Tenth Edition (ICD-10) is the World Health Organization (1994) system. The Diagnostic and Statistical Manual, Fourth Edition, Text Revision (DSM-IV-TR) (American Psychiatric Association 2000) is the North American system, which is widely used in clinical practice and research. These two systems have much in common but there are some variations on specific classifications. The definitions of personality disorder (PD) in both systems refer to *enduring* patterns of interpersonal behaviour (including cognitive and emotional responses) that are *inflexible* and *pervasive* across a *broad range of situations*, and which cause significant *distress* to the individual concerned and/or *social impairment*. Hence, people with PD might suffer personal distress because they cannot achieve their goals and/or might experience social or legal problems even though they might not be distressed about this.

DSM-IV-TR lists ten personality disorders, grouped into three clusters – A, B and C. Cluster A, characterised as the odd or eccentric grouping, includes paranoid, schizoid and schizotypal personality disorders. Cluster B, the dramatic and emotional grouping, includes antisocial, borderline, histrionic and narcissistic personality disorders. Cluster C, the anxiety-based grouping, includes avoidant, dependent and obsessive-compulsive personality disorders. Each PD has a set of seven, eight or nine features which are judged to be present or absent by using a range of interview and collateral data such as case file material and observed behaviour. Where an individual is deemed to exceed the criterion number of these features, they are said to have that particular personality disorder. People may meet the criteria for more than one disorder. Multiple diagnoses tend to fall within the same DSM-IV cluster but some individuals have PDs that cross cluster groupings. For example, antisocial PD (Cluster B), borderline PD (Cluster B) and paranoid PD (Cluster A) are not uncommonly found in forensic mental health settings.

Most theories of personality disorder (PD) recognise core features common to all PDs, namely failure to form adaptive representations of the self and others. Pathology of the self manifests itself in problems with interpersonal boundaries, fragmented representations of others and problems with sense of self and self-regulation. Pathology of interpersonal functioning manifests itself in maladaptive patterns of interpersonal behaviour, difficulties tolerating closeness and intimacy, and problems with collaborative and cooperative relationships.

Personality disorders may or may not be associated with antisocial or violent behaviour. However, the definitions and criteria for some diagnoses, especially those in DSM-IV-TR Cluster B, make this connection much more likely, for example where hostility to others forms part of the diagnostic definition, as in antisocial PD and borderline PD. Some PDs have overlapping criteria between diagnoses, thereby making multiple diagnoses more likely, an issue that will be addressed in the forthcoming DSM-V. Also, since part of the definition of personality disorder is its inflexibility compared with general personality functioning, there is greater potential for those with PD(s) to experience social conflicts and/or distress. The categorical approach to diagnosing PD runs somewhat contrary to general psychological thinking about personality, in which personality traits are seen as continua on which people vary. The diagnostic systems are nevertheless a useful shorthand for considering the range of dysfunctional personality features that an individual may possess and the implications of these for interpersonal functioning and antisocial behaviour.

PSYCHOPATHY

Quite separately from the DSM-IV and ICD-10 classification systems, Hare (1991) researched the concept of psychopathic personality disorder, or psychopathy, developed from Cleckley's (1941) earlier observations in *The Mask of Sanity*. Whilst appearing outwardly intelligent, caring and charming, such individuals turn out to lack empathy and remorse, have egocentric and superficial relationships, and engage in reckless and antisocial behaviour. Hare (1991) developed a reliable system for assessing psychopathy, the Psychopathy Checklist – Revised (PCL-R), which comprises 20 items that are scored on a 3-point scale (0,1 or 2) by reviewing file information such as educational and criminal history together with a structured interview. The 20 items are clustered in terms of 'interpersonal style' (grandiose, superficial and deceitful), 'deficient affective responses' (shallow emotions, callousness, lack of anxiety and lack of remorse), 'irresponsible lifestyle' (including a lack of purposefulness and parasitic lifestyle) and antisocial behaviour (including sensation seeking and impulsive irresponsibility). Psychopathy significantly contributes to predictions of future offending, institutional disruptiveness and difficulty benefiting from conventional treatments. Psychopathy overlaps with but is not identical to DSM-IV-TR Cluster B PDs.

TREATMENT AND MANAGEMENT

How best to provide services for individuals with severe personality disorder who engage in offending behaviour has been a concern of successive governments. In the early 1990s, the Home Office proposed that those classified as meeting the legal criteria for 'Psychopathic Disorder' as defined by the Mental Health Act 1983 should be dealt with through the criminal justice system rather than forensic mental health services. Clinical opposition to this proposal ensured that it was not implemented. The influential 2003 NIMHE report *Personality disorder: No longer a diagnosis of exclusion* (policy implementation guidance for the development of services for people with personality disorder), Department of Health: National Institute for Mental Health in England, stimulated further debate on how best to provide services for PD patients, including forensic patients with various levels of need and risk to others. Subsequently, a joint initiative by the Home Office and Department of Health – the Dangerous and Severe Personality Disorder (DSPD) project – commissioned four pilot treatment centres, two within the Prison Service at HMP Whitemoor and HMP Frankland, and two within the high secure forensic mental health services at Broadmoor and Rampton Hospitals. The aims of the DSPD initiative were increasing public protection, in response to some high-profile violent and sexual offences committed by personality disordered individuals, and improving treatment services for PD offenders within the high secure mental health services (Maden 2007).

SEVERE PERSONALITY DISORDER

Within DSM-IV-TR and ICD-10, individuals might only just exceed the threshold for a disorder or, conversely, might have all of its features, the latter being one characterisation of a 'severe disorder'. Severity might also be seen as the number and range of disorders for which the individual meets the relevant criteria. A third way of thinking about severity is the degree to which the presenting disorder(s) result in major (e.g. rape or homicide) rather than minor (e.g. public nuisance) antisocial behaviours. The last of these concepts was incorporated within the DSPD project, a severe personality disorder being one that is functionally linked to offences from which the victim would find it impossible or very difficult to recover.

There is some evidence linking particular types of PD to particular classes of offending behaviour. Coid (1998) demonstrated links between different types of PD in offender-patients and the functions of violence, for example schizoid PD often being associated with excitement-seeking, while narcissistic PD was associated with seeking to regain control over others. A number of studies have found strong associations between antisocial and/or borderline PDs and violence (e.g. Coid *et al.* 2003). However, different studies have yielded different findings. For clinical assessment and treatment, it is probably more useful to examine links between offending and PDs with individualised formulations rather than seeking global associations.

UNDERLYING PROCESSES

Research has demonstrated a close association between early life experiences and later personality and social development. From the pioneering work of Bowlby (1969, 1973, 1980, 1988) on infants' attachments to their parents and the adverse effects of this being disrupted, research on attachment styles has established that a 'secure' attachment pattern is important for the development of healthy relationships with others in later life. Securely attached children tend to grow up to view both self and others positively, seek closeness and operate in a tolerant and reciprocal fashion. In contrast, disturbed attachments can lead to later personality and relationship problems. Farrington *et al.* (2006) in their long-term prospective study also established that children's exposure to dysfunctional parenting, defined as harsh, erratic or neglectful parenting, was predictive, along with other factors, of later delinquency in boys.

Bartholomew and Horowitz (1991) and Padesky (1995) have shown how early life experiences result in the development of 'schemas' through which individuals view the world and other people, and influence the way in which they seek to relate to others. For example, a schema of self as being 'bad' and others as malevolent can lead to a characteristic way of approaching relationships ('attach and then reject') typical of borderline PD. A self-schema of worthlessness in which others are seen as threatening typically leads to an interactive style of 'compete and dominate', as in narcissistic personality disorder. Because personality disorder is, at its core, a disorder of interpersonal behaviour and relationships, various aspects of the disorder will manifest themselves not only within the individuals' offending behaviour but also within the prison or psychiatric hospital environments to which they may be sent.

BOUNDARIES IN INSTITUTIONAL CARE

Individuals detained in prison and secure hospitals for violence/homicide/sexual offending will, by virtue of their offending, already have broken social and legal boundaries in terms of harming others, and will pose varying levels of risk of doing the same in the institutional setting. Within institutional settings, PD prisoners or patients may present to staff variously as needy, seductive, manipulative or predatory, thereby drawing different reactions from the staff. These may include an urge to self-disclose or hold secrets, to offer favours or special treatment, or to be fearful and distance themselves from engagement with the patient. Some staff may be able to recognise the processes that are unfolding, while others may not and may become drawn deeper into interactions that could become harmful.

Different types of PD influence interpersonal relating in different ways. For example, patients with antisocial PD are likely to push boundaries relating to hospital or prison rules, and engage in self-serving behaviour whilst showing a disregard for the welfare of others. Patients with borderline PD are likely to display fluctuating attachments to other patients and staff, and become highly 'needy' and emotional in their interactions with others. Patients with paranoid PD are likely to be hyper-vigilant for indications of interpersonal threat and react in ways to neutralise those perceived threats, a 'pre-emptive strike'. Patients with narcissistic PD are likely to challenge the rules and good order of an institution by making demands consistent with a style that reinforces their own superiority.

An obvious but important feature of closed environments is that clients and staff spend much longer periods of time together than is the case in outpatient or acute services. Consequently, professional relationships between staff and patients have the potential to become more intense and challenging than in shorter-stay facilities. This provides opportunities for professional relationships to become either too relaxed and personalised or too harsh and punitive, and thereby become subverted into so-called boundary crossings or violations. Within these settings, a boundary crossing might, for example, involve a member of staff inadvertently revealing personal information to a patient that is inappropriate in their role. Some patients may also actively seek out this information, either as a way of feeling closer and special to the staff member (e.g. borderline PD) or as a way of exerting pressure and control on the staff member (antisocial or psychopathic PD).

BOUNDARY VIOLATIONS

It is helpful for staff to be able to distinguish between occasionally inappropriate professional behaviours that do not result in harm (simple boundary crossings) and those which do (boundary violations). Examples of a boundary crossing, in which a member of staff has moved in the direction of a violation but from which the position is recoverable, might be unintentionally revealing personal information or failing to respond appropriately to a patient's legitimate request due to a transient moment of irritation or anger. Boundary crossings can develop into a violation, resulting in damage to others and may also represent a criminal offence. Examples of boundary violations in which serious harm will occur are entering into a physical relationship with a patient or deliberately providing a patient with unauthorised items.

A PD patient's behaviour will differentially interact with a staff member's behaviour in the lead-up to a boundary violation, depending on the staff's own knowledge of personality disorder, the training and supervision they have received, their own personality style and their own personal circumstances. For example, an experienced member of staff whose marriage has broken down, who is leaning increasingly towards work for emotional satisfaction and who has a caring but rather overconfident view of his/her their own capabilities, may recognise that boundary crossings are occurring with a borderline PD patient (e.g. spending more time with the patient than is usual and sharing personal information) but may also feel that (s)he can 'break the rules' and help the patient (as well as fulfilling themselves) through their 'superior knowledge and skills'. Another example might be a junior member of staff who is flattered by the attentions of a seductive patient presenting with psychopathic traits and excited by the possibility of a clandestine relationship. In whatever way boundary violations occur, it is the staff member who holds the duty of care to behave appropriately with the patient and there should therefore be no patient blaming. However, the organisation also has a duty of care to the staff in ensuring that they have been appropriately selected, trained, supervised, monitored and rotated in order to avoid boundary violations.

In summary, where boundary violations occur, particularly the more serious ones such as sexual behaviour or threats to safety and security, these are rarely the result of a single causative factor but rather arise from complex interactions between some or all of the following: (a) over-familiarity between staff and patients due to the close and long-term working environment found within a high secure hospital; (b) negative attitudes, defensive distancing and under-involved/punitive violations, possibly linked to staff burnout; (c) patients' diagnosis and presentation, in particular some manifestations of personality disorder, for example challenge linked to narcissistic traits, neediness linked to borderline traits, and risks of sexual boundary violations with sex offender patients; (d) previous history of boundary violations by staff and/or patients; (e) particular circumstances and experiences of the patient at the time of boundary violation (e.g. positions of relative power or vulnerability at the time); (f) particular circumstances, experiences and vulnerability of the staff member at the time of boundary violation (e.g. marital or financial problems); (g) the capacity of the clinical team and other colleagues to be aware of boundary risks and be supportive of clinical staff; and (h) the ethos of the hospital as an enquiring, supportive and proactive maintainer of appropriate boundaries.

SAFE AND SECURE ENVIRONMENTS

In order to minimise the risk of boundary violations in secure services, a number of preventative measures are prudent. Although boundary violations are a complex interaction between patient, staff and environmental factors, care should be taken at the point of staff selection/appointment to address their awareness of, and attitudes about, professional boundaries, including their likely personal resilience in working with PD patients. Boundary issues should be covered at induction and through regular refresher training. Staff who work with patients who have been assessed as being at particular risk of involvement in boundary violations should be provided with any necessary additional training and supervision. Clinical supervision should include matters such as the time clinicians spend with patients (individually or in groups) and staff members' views on how this is perceived by the patients. Supervision should also encourage exploration of feelings staff may have in relation to their work with patients, and staff should be encouraged to seek support/advice from a manager if they are concerned about interactions between another staff member and any patient(s).

Good multi-disciplinary team-working and facilitated multi-disciplinary reflective practice sessions are also vital for focusing on the role of therapeutic relationships and the maintenance of clear and safe professional boundaries. Security intelligence that can be shared with clinical teams and managers about possible emerging boundary issues is another useful tool for maintaining a safe and healthy environment. Finally, organisations should seek to maintain an open and enquiring stance in relation to learning lessons from things that go wrong or 'near misses' about this important area of work.

All PD patients in secure settings should be assessed to ascertain their likelihood of transgressing boundaries. Patients who are assessed as presenting a significant risk should be subject to a care plan addressing the issues identified and additional specialist care and treatment should be provided as required. Patients should receive information on professional boundaries, including boundary crossings and boundary violations, as part of their care and treatment, which could then be usefully followed up with group sessions to reinforce these messages. These issues will also be key to understanding and working with the patient on wider risk reduction and mental health recovery. A key part of the treatment of patients with PD is the exploration of their relationships with others and the ways this has previously led to problems, including offences. Staff must therefore be helped and supported to work with the ambiguities and subtleties of interpersonal behaviours with PD patients for to withdraw from this would prevent effective treatment.

REFERENCES

Alwin, N., Blackburn, R., Davidson, K., Hilton, M., Logan, C. and Shine, J. (2006) *Understanding Personality Disorder: A Professional Practice Board Report by the British Psychological Society.* Leicester UK: The British Psychological Society.

American Psychiatric Association (2000) *Diagnostic and Statistical Manual of Mental Disorders,* Fourth Edition, Text Revision (DSM-IV-TR). Washington, DC: American Psychiatric Association.

Bartholomew, K. and Horowitz, L.M. (1991) 'Attachment styles among young adults: a test of a four category model.' *Journal of Personality and Social Psychology 61,* 2, 226–244.

Bowlby, J. (1969) *Attachment and loss. Vol. 1: Attachment* (2nd edn). New York: Basic Books.

Bowlby, J. (1973) *Attachment and loss. Vol. 2: Separation: Anxiety and anger.* New York: Basic Books.

Bowlby, J. (1980) *Attachment and loss. Vol. 3: Loss: Sadness and depression.* New York: Basic Books.

Bowlby, J. (1988) *A secure base: Clinical applications of attachment theory.* London: Routledge.

Cleckley, H.M. (1941) *The Mask of Sanity* (1st edition). St Louis: Mosby.

Coid, J. (1998) 'Axis II Disorders and Motivation for Serious Criminal Behaviour.' In A.E. Skodol (ed.) *Psychopathy and Violent Crime.* Washington DC: Academic Psychiatric Press.

Coid, J. (2003) 'Epidemiology, public health and the problem of personality disorder.' *British Journal of Psychiatry 182,* 44, s3–s10.

Farrington, D., Coid, J.W., Harnett, L.M., Jolliffe, D., Soteriou, N., Turner, R.E. and West, D.J. (2006) *Criminal careers up to age 50 and life success up to age 48: new findings from the Cambridge Study in Delinquent Development* (2nd edn). Home Office Research Study 299. Home Office Research, Development and Statistics Directorate, September 2006.

Hare, R.D. (1991) *The Hare Psychopathy Checklist – Revised – Manual.* Toronto: Multi-health Systems.

Livesley, W.J. (ed.) (2000) *Handbook of personality disorders: theory research and ttreatment.* New York: Guilford Press.

Livesley, W.J. (2007) 'The relevance of an integrated approach to the treatment of personality disordered offenders.' *Psychology, Crime and Law 13,* 10, 27–46.

Maden, A. (2007) 'Dangerous and severe personality disorder: antecedents and origins.' *British Journal of Psychiatry 190,* s8–s11.

Padesky, C. (1995) *Mind over mood: Change how you feel by changing the way you think.* New York: Guilford Press.

Chapter 17

MOTHERING ON THE EDGE: BOUNDARY FAILURES IN MATERNAL CARE

Anna Motz

The baby assailed by eyes, ears, nose, skin and entrails all at once, feels it all as one great blooming, buzzing confusion...

William James 1890, p.488

Overview

In this chapter the author describes the dramatic consequences of failures in early maternal care for the infant, and how these are manifested in adulthood. These early experiences adversely impact on the development of individuation, the capacity to tolerate and contain disturbance and the ability to form secure attachments in later life. These profound consequences of early boundary failures are illustrated through clinical material describing maternal narcissism, self-harm and the disavowal of aggression into a violent partner and creation of a toxic relationship.

INTRODUCTION

A central task of the primary carer is to provide a safe, reliable and secure environment in which the baby is able, eventually, to make sense of this 'blooming, buzzing confusion' that threatens to overwhelm her. The development of the perceptual apparatus is part of what makes the world meaningful, but in order for the baby's sense of herself to develop alongside trust in the external world there needs to be the presence of reliable, sensitive care-takers. When this is absent the sense of great confusion may continue throughout later life. This chapter explores three different types of boundary failures in mothering, and the serious harm these cause.

The first boundary failure I describe is one where the mother cannot see the baby as a separate person, but rather thinks of her as part of herself, making no distinction between them. This disturbance is often intergenerational, mirroring how, in their early lives, these women's own mothers treated them as narcissistic extensions of themselves. Welldon (1988) describes this as a perversion of motherhood, and identifies this transgenerational transmission of objectification as central to maternal child abuse.

The second type of boundary failure is found within a toxic partnership, in which each partner projects significant aspects of themselves onto the other, and disowns them; the unprotective mother pairs with a violent partner. In these relationships the man carries her aggression and she identifies with the vulnerable, helpless infant aspect of him.

The third manifestation of boundary failure is often demonstrated through self-harm. When there has been neglect or abuse by the mother (usually the primary caregiver) or carer in early life, the infant is left without what can be thought of as psychic skin. The requisite process for this development is described below, and its failure leaves the infant without a sense of what is inside or outside herself, a frightening state that can lead to abuses of her body in order to create a sense of boundaries and cohesion.

After birth the infant cannot differentiate between what is outside and what is inside herself, and desperately requires holding by the mother, in order to have a sense of being contained and integrated. In order to develop primary integration, that is, a sense of internal coherence, what Winnicott calls 'the indwelling of the psyche in the soma' (Winnicott 1960, p.589), the mother has to provide a reliable, consistent and responsive environment for the baby. This is akin to Bion's notion of containment by the mother of the infant and is crucial for the development of thinking, of a sense of being held together and not just being in a state of 'nameless dread' in which no sense can be made of the terrifying forces of hunger, rage and fear, and no containment is offered that enables the needs to be met and the feelings to be named. This postnatal infant idyll is well captured in Bick's (1968) image of:

> ...the nipple in the mouth together with the holding and talking and familiar smelling mother... (p.484)

In due course the infant internalises a feeling of an 'amniotic sac inside', a secure boundary or 'psychic skin' that separates self and other, inside and outside (Bick 1968; Winnicott 1960).

If this holding mother, who can bear the force of her infant's primitive needs, and enable her to develop a psychic skin, a sense of a boundaried self, is absent, or only inconsistently available, the infant will develop what Bick calls a secondary skin in its place. As the infant develops she finds it difficult, if not impossible, to know where her own boundaries are located. The sense of an embodied self is seriously distorted. This can lead to eating disorders and self-harm in adolescence and adulthood as she attempts to create boundaries and contain the force of unmanageable conflicts and feelings through concrete action on the body. The marks she leaves on her body when she self-harms are the expression of earlier trauma, and its attempted mastery.

THE BABY IN THE MIND

Women who were maltreated or neglected in early life often have particular difficulties in forming attachments with their children, despite their desperate wishes not to repeat the destructive patterns of their own lives. Their ability to relate to their babies as separate from them can be profoundly impaired. This inability to think of the baby as an individual can begin in pregnancy where s/he is not thought of as a separate human developing within the mother, but either as a grotesque intrusion or an undifferentiated part of her, with no distinct borders. Some women become preoccupied with a sense of invasion by an alien being, and make efforts to get rid of it, either mentally or physically, revealing their unconscious terrors about the unborn baby.

The baby, in the mother's mind, can sometimes assume the form of an idealised maternal creature, who will herself offer perfect care and love to the mother. The birth of the actual baby, with its demands, needs and rages, can be experienced as awful. Through her psychoanalytic work with women who were pregnant, new mothers, or facing fertility difficulties, Pines (1993) repeatedly observed the tremendous disappointment that actually giving birth causes in women who longed for fullness, care and mothering during their pregnancy.

The extent of disturbance in some can be akin to a psychotic experience and, indeed, the whole sense of where one body and self begins and ends, and where another starts, can be highly confusing and disorienting, particularly so for women who have not been given a sense of themselves as integrated wholes, but who have for much of their early lives been treated as part objects by their own mothers and carers. A clinical illustration of this comes from a heavily pregnant young woman who repeatedly inserted wire coat hangers into her vagina, hoping to hook her baby out and see what was inside her, feeling so frightened of invasion from within. This reflected her fears of her own reproductive system and a real inability to symbolise, or to recognise the possibility of a separate human being who could grow inside her. She felt so filled with poisonous feelings and primitive anxieties that she believed she would turn any new life inside her bad. Her conscious reason for wanting to see the baby was for reassurance, to see evidence of the real baby inside her, but her unconscious reasons were connected to both suicidal and murderous feelings. She had no human baby in her mind and she could not imagine one inside her body. Her actions were dangerous and destructive, a form of self-harm. Additionally she had a long history of cutting, both on and inside her body through inserting glass and other objects, and in one way it seemed that harming her baby would simply be an extension of that self-mutilation. She was clearly attacking her reproductive body and the baby it had produced.

In fantasy the pregnancy offers both physical and psychic promises of an all-encompassing holding, becoming in imagination a kind of re-birth for the mother herself. In such cases one can see how the mother struggles with her pregnancy, and its reality, as opposed to fantasised elements involving extreme idealisation (the transcendent baby mother) or denigration (monstrous parasitical creature.)

The stark reality of the actual birth, and the evidence of separateness of a real infant, can be experienced as brutal and wholly unwanted by these desperate young women. Not only are their own fantasies of being loved and cared for shattered, but also they are faced with harsh evidence of their own impoverished capacity to nurture and comfort, feeling persecuted and helpless in the face of relentless demands. The baby's cries echo their own unmet needs and are intolerable to bear.

ATTACHMENT PATTERNS

Women who have disturbed early relationships with mothers and other caretakers are at increased risk of developing other difficulties in emotional regulation and relationships, finding the demands of intimacy intolerable. They are in a high-risk group for developing difficulties within intimate relationships and may later be classified as having borderline personality disorder, on the basis of features like impulsivity, self-harm, eating disorders, and tremendous fear of closeness, alternating with terror of abandonment. When they have their own babies they face significant difficulties in seeing their children as separate from them, providing consistent and reliable care and protecting them from repeated experiences of neglect and abuse that tragically mirror their own. This is often in stark contrast to conscious wishes to spare their children the deprivation and abuse of their own early lives, reflecting the power of unconscious forces and non-verbal early experiences.

Many mothers with borderline personality disorder (BPD) have a fundamental difficulty in acknowledging the independent psychological existence of the infant and are motivated by their own unresolved traumatic attachment issues. The traumatised parent may re-traumatise their infant through insensitive, inconsistent, frightening and confusing interactions (Beebe and Lachman 1988).

> The parent with BPD is often unable to put their distress into words. They are frequently consumed with frustration and anger and have difficulty with the range and intensity of emotions that are aroused in a relationship with a dependent infant... The mother may fluctuate in her perception of the infant, as a 'good' part of the parent's self to be protected from abuse or as the 'bad' part of the self that deserved to be abused. At other times, the infant becomes the persecutor, the original 'bad' parent and is attacked. (Newman and Stevenson 2005, p.388)

Clinical illustration

Jay was charged with cruelty and neglect after her six-month-old daughter was battered to death by her partner. She was 18 and had an extensive history of trauma in her own life, and little sense of her own self-worth, having been violently and sexually abused by her stepfather and neglected by her mother, who appeared to have 'turned a blind eye' to her daughter's vulnerability and the sexual violence to which she was subjected. Jay had become pregnant to an older partner when she was 16. The baby, a girl, had been born prematurely and her survival was in doubt from the beginning of her tragically short life. Jay was now pregnant with a second child, some 18 months after her daughter's death, and wanted to assure social services that she had matured sufficiently to protect and nurture this new child. I was asked to assess whether or not this was, in fact, the case.

She had pleaded guilty to the charges that had been pressed against her, and had eventually been convicted for neglect but the charge of cruelty had been dropped. In his summing up, the judge expressed the strong sense that she had suffered enough through the death of her child, and that her main crime was to allow her violent partner to have unlimited and unsupervised access to a highly vulnerable infant, rather than to have wilfully committed acts of ill-treatment herself.

My encounter with Jay was painful. She remained largely unresponsive throughout two assessment sessions and gave only the briefest of answers to questions. I was left with the strong impression that she was somehow deadened, and had been emotionally petrified since early life. She was frozen, unreachable and almost mute.

Her own mother had been distant and neglectful and one of Jay's wishes was to have a daughter herself. When we explored what she had hoped for, it became clear that unconsciously she had wished for a little girl with whom she could merge in a blissful state of union, as she imagined other mothers achieved with their daughters. She longed to feel fulfilled and loved and had, in pregnancy, experienced this sense. Birth had shattered this for her and she felt even emptier than before.

Despite her raw vulnerability it was hard to reach her and my usual sense of wanting to take care of, or rescue, the desperate child within was absent in my counter-transference to her. I realised, after close reflection, that this mirrored her own profound difficulty in taking care of another, that her frozen state and apparent dissociation both protected and removed her from the world. All caretaking, of herself or an infant, had stopped before it began.

It seemed that her own rage had gone underground, and that rather than express her aggressive impulses, which she feared might completely overwhelm her, she found herself locked into a familiar relationship where her apparent protector had continually abused and hurt her, even threatening her with death. She had one close confidante in a former foster carer, who had advised her to leave this man, but she felt she needed him above anyone else. The question was why she had chosen this particular partner, why she had remained with him; and the tragedy was how fully she had abdicated all control of her own body and mind, and colluded unconsciously in her baby's murder. Could any of this be made conscious?

The risks of addressing her disavowal of aggression were significant. Her conception of herself as helpless in the face of her partner's demands was psychologically protective for her, and her own responsibility for allowing him to 'take care' of her daughter, whom she had found covered with bruises after one occasion when he had been on his own with her, were protective, in that they shielded her from the crippling levels of guilt that the child's death had left her with. Confronting her sense of herself as victim could result in the onset of severe depression, but not doing so would leave her stuck. I considered it urgent that Jay should be helped to see how her own unarticulated rage had contributed to her choice of partner, her passivity in the face of an unplanned pregnancy and her emotionally petrified state. Her unconscious response to her daughter's fragility and prematurity had been to distance herself, rather than face up to the helplessness that she saw so concretely and painfully reflected in her infant.

What would it take to address this protective but ultimately ineffectual defence? How could one recommend rehabilitation of a child to the care of a woman who was, in an essential way, complicit in the death of her first child? She had made repeated suicide attempts herself after her daughter's death, making the most serious attempt during the period of time when she awaited sentencing, showing how fragile she was, and how hard it was to contain feelings of grief and guilt. She repeatedly said that she felt that she had already died, that she too had been killed when her daughter had been, seeing herself in that battered infant.

This tragic case of a failure to establish boundaries between the mother and her infant, and to respond protectively to the essential needs of the baby for safety, demonstrates how suicidal feelings in a young mother can also lead to a situation in which homicidal impulses are enacted, even if not by the woman herself, but, as in this case, through the actions of her violent partner. The earlier boundary failure within Jay's psychic development was her inability to acknowledge and manage her own destructive and aggressive impulses that tended to be disowned, and projected into her violent partner. He carried this violence for her, and she in turn was able to disavow it, remaining forever the passive victim. This psychic splitting had been essential for her survival in early life when she did not trust herself to express rage at either the stepfather who abused her or the mother who turned away, being hopelessly dependent on them. Indeed, even in discussion with me she could only express anger at her stepfather, retaining an idealised view of her mother as helpless and innocent, despite the cruelty she had allowed Jay to suffer.

The question of Jay's depression, and also her unacknowledged rage, was central. She needed to be shown how much she identified with the damaged and dying baby. Perhaps part of the fantasy in relation to her firstborn baby was that if she was hurt, even killed, the part of her that was so damaged could also be killed off. At the same time she was unaware of this. This dynamic can be understood as an unconscious one, and can also be seen in the psychological state known as 'learned helplessness' in that the mother perceives herself as incapable of taking protective action, for herself or her child. Ultimately she is fused with the helpless infant and cannot bear this awareness, facing the choice of either violently turning away from this hated part of herself, allowing it to be killed, or killing herself directly. It seemed that this young woman attempted to do both, alternating between one and the other option, but that what she was not able to do was to enlist any lively or protective capacities to rescue both her infant and herself from a situation of domestic terrorism.

In assessment she was already 'as if' dead. Furthermore, without intensive treatment to build up her ability to face the horror of what she had allowed to happen, the risk of repeating the pattern remained high. That is, there was a high likelihood that she would be drawn to violent partners, and see the baby as part of herself, deserving poor treatment and impossible to protect.

SKIN AND ITS CONTAINMENT

From earliest infancy skin and its sensations are central to the emotional experience of the baby, who is held against her mother's breast, nursed, caressed, tickled and bathed. It is through touch that important early bonds are formed before the baby has language or the ability to conceptualise the world. For some babies the experience of being undressed, with its exposure of skin to air, and the sense of being unravelled, is itself an attacking, disintegrating event, and for almost all, comfort is derived from skin-to-skin contact with mother and the experience of being put down, away from her, is distressing, causing them to cry. The psychological evidence for the significance of skin-to-skin contact in early bonding is robust,[1] and the analytic literature asserts the primacy of early experience in providing the foundations for the construction of an integrated self.[2]

For babies who have not had the reliable presence of a mother holding them, both physically and psychologically – the bodily sensation of being held, fed, bathed, soothed and having their needs met – there is a dramatic impact on their sense of internal integration. It is evident that from infancy, integration starts from the outside in – physical containment is required for psychic containment and is essential in the development of a coherent sense of self, and ultimately in the construction of a perception of internal and external, a notion of one's own mind and body, demarcated clearly. The body ego, as Freud (1923) termed it, is the first ego, and disruptions in its care have a significant impact on the development of the psychic structures, the ego or the sense of self in mediation with the external world.

Skin is the boundary, the protective shield that separates self and other but also the point of contact with another and the line between inside and outside, the surface onto which sensation is felt. It is boundary, site of perception and

---

1   Regardless of their theoretical position, many scientists and paediatricians are convinced that touch and close bodily contact are necessary conditions for the infant's normal and healthy development (Grossmann, Thane and Grossmann 1981).

2   'In its most primitive form the parts of the personality are felt to have no binding force amongst themselves and must therefore be held together in a way that is experienced by them passively, by the skin functioning as a boundary… The stage of primal splitting…can now be seen to rest on this earlier process of containment of self and object by their respective skins' (Bick 1968, p.484).

point of impact. The connections between disorders of the skin and early attachment experiences are central to understanding both the development and meaning of self-harm.

Clinical illustration: Self-harm and boundary failure

Maya was a woman in her early twenties when she was referred to me for psychotherapy. She had a history of upheaval and trauma in her childhood. She was the youngest of three girls, had never known her father, and had been largely neglected by her mother, who was herself in her late teens when she gave birth to Maya, in Eastern Europe. She had travelled with her mother and older sisters from country to country, where her mother formed various short-lived, often violent, relationships until eventually settling in England.

When Maya was 19, despite taking birth control pills, she became pregnant by her partner of a few months, who was some eleven years older than her. She felt weak and faint during her pregnancy and was convinced, at times, that she was at risk of death. Throughout this unplanned pregnancy she tried to poison her unborn baby and herself through ingesting bleach. She also seriously considered shooting herself in the head, as she believed this to be potentially less harmful to the baby, seeming to deny the intrinsic link between her own life and her baby's survival. On the one hand she saw her unborn daughter as part of herself, on the other saw her as a kind of immortal, transcendent being who would emerge unscathed from her dead body. This was a delusional attack on reality, and a massive denial of the depths of her own destructiveness, and the link between her homicidal and suicidal urges.

By swallowing bleach she said she hoped to drown herself and her unborn child in a way that would also leave them 'pure in death'. She understood this to be a suicidal wish but could not consider it as attempted murder too, feeling so persecuted by the child who grew inside her, and whom she felt was not fully alive.

Through making cuts on her own body Maya had found a way to manage the inchoate feelings of despair that often overwhelmed her; after cutting she tended to the wounds and this offered her a form of self-mothering of which she had been deprived in early life. Significantly, her self-harm during pregnancy alerted the child protection services to her own unmet needs, and to the risk that she could pose to herself and her unborn baby. She was referred for treatment in a therapeutic residential unit where she was able to engage in both individual and group therapy and to be cared for in her own right, finally in receipt of the maternal containment she longed for. Here she finally found an opportunity for her sense of deprivation and rage to be addressed, and in these conditions her pregnancy was able to continue in a safe and secure way through to birth.

When the baby was born she was greatly relieved that it was a boy, as this helped her see how different he was from her, and gave her a sense of triumph and wonder about what her own body could produce. She was, with the help of the therapeutic residential placement, able to establish a sense of separateness between him and herself, and to develop a real attachment to him. She was still terrified of being left alone, and when he left to be cared for by others, even for short periods of time, her own feelings of vulnerability intensified, though she was able in time to overcome these fears, and to use the therapeutic holding offered to her. She became able to respond to his cries without feeling overwhelmed by her own sense of need, and sadness, and was delighted that she could comfort him, sometimes by simply holding him, or speaking to him, without actually feeding him. She learned about her own capacity for containment, and her own need for care, and began to articulate rather than enact on her body, giving up the cutting that had sustained her for so long.

There was some hope that through the therapeutic care she received within a residential setting, she could offer her infant son the experience of a maternal holding environment he required. Maya's case illustrates how self-harm can be seen as an attempt to create boundaries and order for herself to overcome a developmental trauma she had experienced in her own infancy, with a mother who could not provide this sense of an 'amniotic sac' inside, and ease the transition from birth to earliest life. It also shows how, despite this failure in her own infancy, women can develop the capacity to provide a different experience for their own children, though this may not come 'naturally' but have to be developed and nurtured within a therapeutic situation that offers them 'holding' and containment.

DISCUSSION

This chapter has explored the kinds of boundary violations that underlie both self-harm and child abuse. Often crimes that women commit are not detected because of secrecy and because the targets are their own bodies or those of their children, who may keep silent about this abuse. When women abuse the children, with whom they identify narcissistically, they are re-creating patterns of boundary violations from their own early lives. Their children's bodies and minds are not seen as precious, separate and individual, but as distorted mirrors of themselves. In sexual and physical abuse of children their bodies are used for the gratification of the mother's own need for triumph and revenge, often against her own cruel parents, and can also be understood as an expression of her own self-hatred.

Mothers fail to protect their child from a violent partner for various reasons, including their own difficulties in accepting or addressing the damage that is being done. In some cases they are themselves so humiliated and intimidated by their partners that they have given up the possibility of protecting either their children or themselves.

In this chapter I have also described how in some extreme cases of couple abuse of children, projective identification of all aggression and cruelty is located into one partner, often the man, which allows the woman to disavow her feelings of rage and hatred. She, meanwhile, becomes the apparent receptacle of all weakness and vulnerability; and within the couple this psychotic split is maintained, and both mother and child can be harmed irrevocably. Throughout their relationship the main currency of communication is violence and the threat of violence. This was evident in the clinical illustration of Jay, a depressed, 'frozen' young woman locked into a violent relationship where her daughter was eventually killed.

In other cases mothers identify so completely with the helpless and vulnerable child that they cannot bear to acknowledge what is happening and the harm that this child is suffering. Powerful and primitive mechanisms like denial and projective identification protect the mother from facing the damage that is being done, often until there is external intervention, including childcare proceedings, when she may herself feel blamed and accused. At one level she accepts responsibility for turning a blind eye to facts she couldn't face seeing, but at another she feels that she can't be blamed for this, as her own experiences of trauma, and abuse, and her own sense of her child as a part of her, makes this turning away inevitable. How could she have done otherwise? This is the work of therapy with those mothers who choose to try to address this painful question.

Women can both enact and enable cruelty against their own children. In cases where the boundaries between themselves and their children are distorted, often repeating their own pattern of being narcissistically treated by their mothers, these women see their children as aspects of themselves, to be treated with the same contempt and disregard they feel they themselves deserve, and to which they have become accustomed. In this way the mother enacts her worst fear, and treats her own child as she was herself treated, that is, neglected and abused. This is against all her conscious wishes and hopes. Such is the tragedy and force of the repetition compulsion. The task of forensic psychotherapists and child care professionals is to identify these forces, so often unconscious and shameful to bear, and to help the mothers themselves to recognise them, and offer them intensive help to understand, control and finally alter these entrenched patterns of relating.

REFERENCES

Beebe, B. and Lachman, F.M. (1988) 'Mother-infant mutual influence and precursors of psychic structure.' In A. Goldberg (ed.), *Progress in Self Psychology*, Vol. 3, pp. 3-25. Hillsdale, NJ: Analytic Press.

Bick, E. (1968) 'The Experience of Skin in Early Object Relations.' In M. Harris Williams (ed.) (1987) *Collected Papers of Martha Harris and Esther Bick*. Perthshire: Clunie Press.

Freud, S. (1923) *The Ego and the Id*. SE XIX.

Grossmann, K., Thane, K. and Grossmann, K.E. (1981) 'Maternal tactual contact of the newborn after various postpartum conditions of mother-infant contact.' *Developmental Psychology 17*, 158–169.

James, W. (1957) *The Principles of Psychology: Volume One*. London: Dover Publications.

Motz, A. (2008) *The Psychology of Female Violence: Crimes Against the Body* (2nd edn). Hove: Brunner-Routledge.

Newman, L. and Stevenson, C. (2005) 'Ghosts in the Nursery: Parenting and Borderline Personality Disorder.' *Clinical Child Psychology and Psychiatry 10*, 3, 385–394.

Pines, D. (1993) *A Woman's Unconscious Use of Her Body*. London: Virago.

Welldon, E. (1988) *Mother, Madonna, Whore: The Idealisation and Denigration of Motherhood*. New York: Guilford Press.

Winnicott, D.W. (1960) 'The Theory of the Infant–Parent Relationship'. *Journal of Psycho-Analysis 41*. Reprinted in *The Maturational Processes and the Facilitating Environment*. Hogarth Press, 1965/Karnac Books, 1990.

Chapter 18

BOUNDARY MATTERS IN A FORENSIC LEARNING DISABILITY SERVICE

Richard Curen

Overview

This chapter attempts to make connections between society's aggressive and negative attitudes towards people with learning disabilities and the complex nature and manifestation of boundary ruptures in the consulting room. The way that we as a society treat people with learning disabilities, in the street, in our benefits and legal systems, and in our use of language, all emerges in our clinics and in the way we engage. Starting with a discussion of the shocking revelations that came out of the Winterbourne View scandal and previous institutional abuse cases, the chapter makes links between features of assessment and treatment of forensic patients attending a community-based clinic and some of the psychoanalytic theories that help shed light on this work. The chapter ends by concluding that it is essential to define the boundary before a boundary transgression can take place. Therapeutic work with people who find they have retreated into autistic states, owing to boundary violations or a lack of environmental containment, for whatever reason, needs time and energy in order to be able to make good use of the therapeutic process.

INTRODUCTION

I start this chapter by discussing the current plight of some people with learning disabilities, specifically those deemed to have 'challenging behaviours'. In May

2011 the BBC's Panorama programme broadcast an undercover documentary that highlighted the abuse and consequent suffering of patients living in an assessment and treatment centre called Winterbourne View. According to the BBC (2011):

> During five weeks spent filming undercover, Panorama's reporter captured footage of some of the hospital's most vulnerable patients being repeatedly pinned down, slapped, dragged into showers while fully clothed, taunted and teased.

The screening and subsequent media interest reignited the debate about the institutional care of people with learning disabilities and especially those people with 'challenging behaviour'. Questions were raised in the House of Commons and the House of Lords about the Care Quality Commission, who are charged with inspecting these settings, as well as the systemic failures within the organisation that employed the 11 implicated members of staff, a number of whom have been charged with, but not yet found guilty of, the ill-treatment of patients under the Mental Health Act. What I hope to show in this chapter is that the extreme boundary violations that took place in Winterbourne View are enactments of unconscious hatred of people with learning disabilities.

Winterbourne was not an isolated occurrence (for example Longcare in 1994, Cornwall Partnership NHS Trust in 2006, Sutton and Merton Primary Care NHS Trust in 2007) and was of course met with righteous indignation by all those who watched the programme. However, these high-profile incidents do not tell the whole story. Every day people with learning disabilities are subjected to both overt and covert attacks from others on the street and in their homes. What was so shocking in the BBC programme was the often sadistic violence. There was outrage at what the perpetrators did, outrage about the systemic failures, and empathy for the victims and the victims' families, who wrongly believed that their loved ones were being cared for. But is it any wonder that some people do inflict both physical and psychological attacks on this group of people? We can see examples of harassment and hatred throughout history: the medieval fool who was beaten, mocked and laughed at; the Victorian freak shows; the Nazis in Germany. Hitler described disabled people as useless eaters unworthy of life. The eugenics movement has much to answer for, in particular the underlying fear still pervading our society today of the dependency of people with learning disabilities and the drain they may make on our resources and on each of us personally.

The National Council for Civil Liberties (NCCL) (1951), in their pamphlet on the treatment of mental health patients, states that people with learning disabilities are an:

...integral part of the human race; their existence constitutes an unspoken demand on us. The extent to which we guard their right to the fullest and most useful life, the extent to which we guarantee to them the maximum freedom which they can enjoy and the extent to which we help their families to give them the love they need is a measure of the extent to which we ourselves are civilized. (p.40)

Pring (2011) writes in his book on the Longcare care scandal that it was difficult for people to understand how the abuse there had gone on for so long, and wonders why no one could understand why the residents hadn't confided in their families. He goes on to say that the sad reason was because the message they had imbibed for so long was that they were not deserving of the same rights as other people. The same can be said for those individuals we saw in Winterbourne View and in the interviews with the parents. Those who did try to alert their families could not make themselves understood. Their reluctance to return was seen as a wish to stay at home at the end of an enjoyable weekend. They were said to be 'playing up'. Others were too scared to do anything but nod and force a grin when asked if everything was alright.

More recently an Equality and Human Rights Commission (EHRC) (2011) report into disability-related harassment found that:

- Cases reported in the media are simply the 'tip of the iceberg'.

- Harassment is commonplace, with many people with learning disabilities believing it is inevitable.

- People with learning disabilities often do not report crimes.

- Systemic failures exist in public authorities to recognise the extent and impact of harassment.

The report ends by recommending that what is needed is a transformation of the way disabled people are viewed, valued and included in society. This is especially true of those forensic individuals who challenge services and challenge our own limits and boundaries.

A PLETHORA OF DIAGNOSES

I will now attempt to highlight some of the boundary issues that have emerged in clinical work at Respond[1] with patients with learning disabilities who have

---

1   Respond is a voluntary sector organisation based in central London. It provides assessment and psychotherapeutic treatment services to children and adults with learning disabilities who have experienced abuse or trauma, as well as those with various offending behaviours.

experienced abuse and have abused others. Boundaries – whether those of the victims or the perpetrators – are *prima facie* the main reasons that people are referred to the clinic where I work. Patients come with a multitude of diagnoses, with a large number each having a complex mixture of learning disabilities, mental health problems, Autistic Spectrum Disorder (ASD) and Attention Deficit Hyperactivity Disorder (ADHD). This is almost always coupled with a history of victimisation and often with a history of being violent towards themselves and/or others. This group are often considered to be hard to treat due to misunderstandings about their ability to engage in psychotherapeutic treatment. Intellectual ability was for many years an essential prerequisite for treatability and it wasn't until the early 1980s, and the pioneering work of clinicians such as Alvarez (1992) and Sinason (1989, 1992, 1994), that *emotional ability* became an important yardstick of treatability.

Sinason (1992) pioneered the idea of a 'secondary handicap' as a feature that is employed by people with learning disabilities as a defence against trauma, and as a way to also cover up the primary handicap. Corbett (2009) introduced the concept of 'disability transference' where a disabled patient projects unbearable feelings into the therapist. With these concepts in mind it is possible to start to make sense of the experience of psychotherapy with people with learning disabilities. People with ASD, learning disabilities and ADHD are most often characterised as having increased levels of impulsivity, or a deficit in internal inhibitors, a lack of empathy and often do not read social cues or familiar boundary conventions. Not knowing where one ends and where others begin is a feature that reoccurs not simply in some of Respond's patients but also in people suffering from psychosis and those with personality disorders. What makes this client group different is the combination of diagnostic features that intersect with and affect each other and the way they manifest in relation to the outside world.

THE CASE OF MR C[2]

Mr C was referred for a forensic risk assessment. He was 17 and had a moderate learning disability, ASD and ADHD. He lived with his parents and had a history of challenging behaviours from the age of seven. He seemed to have little concern for danger and pain and would regularly jump off high walls, from his moving bicycle and down the stairs. As with other young men with these diagnoses, Mr C and his family had received support from the local Child

---

2   All of the case studies in this paper use initials unrelated to the actual individual in order to maintain confidentiality.

and Adolescent Mental Health Service. The family did not engage for long, wanting to avoid administering the recommended medication and wishing also to deal with any problems 'in house'. This had led to a stand-off between the school and the family, with behaviours only being reported at the school and the family insisting that Mr C's behaviour at home was not a problem. Mr C was considered to be a risk to himself and his fellow students, as well as to members of staff. He had been violent towards staff and pupils, including threats to kill, and had displayed sexually inappropriate behaviour towards female staff by asking them intimate details about their relationships and by transgressing people's personal space, especially from behind. He touched the necks of female staff at the school and would push or try to pin them against a wall or desk.

During the assessment it became evident that Mr C was very limited in his understanding of appropriate boundaries and his sexual knowledge was also very limited. The assessment took place over 12 weeks and in the sessions Mr C called the assessor 'Mr Penis-head' in a taunting and childlike manner. He kicked the walls while lounging on the couch, not stopping when asked to do so, but carrying on using slightly less force in a very provocative way. He laughed uncontrollably and clapped his hands in a very autistic manner. Any mention of sex or drugs and Mr C worked himself into a frenzy of clapping and laughing that was very difficult, but not impossible, for him to come down from. This pushing of boundaries made the assessment sessions particularly difficult for the assessor but quite straightforward in terms of the assessment needing to find out about Mr C's sexual knowledge and about his ability to control himself. Mr C's infantile understanding of sex, coupled with his aggressive tendencies, was an unpredictable and potentially explosive mix. It was a challenge not to let him get under the skin of the assessor. His *modus operandi* was to intimidate and push himself into those around him; calling the assessor Mr Penis-head was a way of putting his penis into the assessor's mind. Mr C sometimes became sexually aroused during the sessions and was simultaneously excited and confused by this. The effect on the assessor was to feel attacked and want to turn away from him. However, similarly to Mr C, the assessor felt unable to think. How could this be understood, how could what the therapist experiences be related to the patient without being attacked again straight away? It was as if he was being violated by this young man who was testing the boundaries of the assessment/therapeutic space. In order to try to help Mr C to regulate himself, the assessor found that talking about animals, especially horses, and the loss of a loved one, seemed to calm the patient significantly and the patient was then better able to reflect on his worries about who he was and why he was being assessed.

Confronting this situation at the clinic, the assessor was able to make use of supervision that concentrated on the impact on himself and the potential meanings of that, as well as how to approach the work. Although this was a time-limited assessment, the assessor used the transference and his counter-transference reactions to make sense of the material being presented. Meltzer (1994) states in his paper on adolescent confusional states:

> …that the analyst needs to provide containment and shielding as well as take on the ego-function of thinking, spending his time not in seeking new material but, rather, in reviewing and bringing order into the previous events and material of the analysis. (p.457)

The assessor therefore provides the scaffolding during the session, using the awareness of the developing therapeutic relationship. Mr C seemed to feel contained by seeing and hearing the assessor trying to make sense of the phenomenological experience of being in the room together and was able to think about the confusional states that emerged during the sessions.

I have written previously (Curen 2009) that many abused and traumatised patients seen at Respond have internalised the idea of a protective shell in order to protect themselves from further abandonments like those experienced in childhood. Previous experiences of separation and loss mean that issues of relating to others are combined with feelings of anxiety and of depression. In the case of sex offenders with learning disabilities a 'solution' to these internal conflicts is to employ sexualisation, which converts aggression to sadism (Campbell 1989; Glasser 1996). The intention to unconsciously destroy those people that have abandoned them is then converted into a wish to hurt and control that is acted out on their victims. I shall illustrate this with another case study.

THE CASE OF MR D

Mr D was a 47-year-old man with a moderate learning disability and ASD, who had sexually assaulted a number of young boys and been seen masturbating in public on a number of occasions. He was referred for psychotherapeutic treatment, which lasted four years. His history was one of abandonment and sexual abuse. At the age of two months Mr D was given up by his mother and lived in care for the rest of his life. He was diagnosed with ASD and 'mental retardation'. He was often seen self-harming via head-banging and would also occasionally attack staff. At 13 he was sent to a mainstream school but was found to be too difficult. He was sexually abused by a male foster carer during his teenage years. He was seen masturbating in public during his adolescence and this continued until his early 20s. He then sexually assaulted a number of young boys with whom he had contact via a local Scout group.

Mr D presented in sessions as keen to engage but only to a limited degree. He did not want to talk about the offences, choosing instead to fill the room with ceaseless chatting. He ignored the therapist's interpretations, choosing to 'run' the sessions. The moderate learning disability and accompanying ASD might have meant that he struggled to allow the therapist into his world. The therapist often felt deskilled and unable to access the emotional world of Mr D. However, another way to make contact was via the transference experience. Mr D often sat with his hand underneath his crossed legs, as if he was trying to get his hand between his buttocks and into his anus. He would then remove his hand and enjoy smelling and exploring his fingers, often biting and picking the dead skin from around his fingernails and eating it. This behaviour was hard to stomach and although this was pointed out to him, he continued nonetheless. The therapist asked himself if this was an unconscious attack on him, or did he mean to try and elicit feelings of disgust in order to give the therapist a sense of how he felt about himself? It was certainly hard to think clearly while this was happening in the room as the feelings of disgust were often quite overwhelming.

However, what first appears as an attack could also be a self-soothing and comforting activity. Ogden (2008) describes a patient who refused to bathe and whose intense body odour would accompany him everywhere. Ogden initially felt invaded by the patient, like he was getting under his skin. He later became aware of the patient's projective identification engendering in him feelings of being painfully invaded 'by his internal object mother' (p.226). The therapist also experienced Mr D's behaviour as invasive, but it is possible to see it as a feature of the disability transference. Mr D felt that his mother had abandoned him when she realised that he had a learning disability. The rejection and subsequent sexual abuse cast a shadow over all of his encounters. He had witnessed many carers coming to help him and then leaving him, and this repetition of the trauma of his mother's abandonment precipitated a retreat into secondary handicap functioning and pathological autism.

The next case study continues the theme of boundary phenomena and the need for therapists to tune into the transference and counter-transference in the sessions.

THE CASE OF MR A

Mr A was 58 at the time of the referral and was referred by his social worker. He had a mild learning disability and ASD. He had recently been found guilty of a sexual assault on a 13-year-old boy. He was awaiting sentencing and was later given a conditional discharge. He was originally referred for a 12-week risk assessment, but it was decided that psychotherapeutic treatment would be more appropriate given that some areas of risk were already known and that the treatment would include regular reports that would assess levels of risk.

Mr A was brought up at home by his parents until he was eight, at which point his mother left home. Mr A believed that she continued to live locally but had never seen her again. Mr A was sexually abused by his father from the age of nine until his father died when Mr A was in his early teens. He then went to live with some relatives but got into trouble with the police for burglary and stealing from cars. He was convicted of various offences and spent some time in prison. There were no other recorded contacts with the police, but there was information relating to other incidents involving males (not minors) held on Social Services files. It was stated on file that there were difficulties placing Mr A in a family setting due to 'homosexual tendencies'. It was also noted that Mr A might need counselling on account of obsessive behaviour regarding a male friend. At one point the torn underpants of another resident were found in Mr A's bed. There was also an allegation made by another resident in a care home that Mr A had pushed him onto a bed and touched him between the legs.

It was alleged in the index offence that Mr A put his hands down the front and back of a 13-year-old boy, touching his penis and bottom. The incident took place after a period in which Mr A and the boy had had regular contact, often saying hello in the mornings as Mr A visited a café next to the newspaper shop which the boy did his paper round from. The relationship developed as they both shared an interest in and supported a local football team. Mr A offered to give the boy some football programmes. The offence is said to have occurred one morning as Mr A handed over the football programmes.

Mr A attended a psychotherapy assessment and was assessed by a member of the clinical team. Mr A was not clear why he was there. It was suggested that it had something to do with people being concerned about him, particularly after the incident with the paperboy. He denied the offence ever took place and resented having to attend treatment as part of the conditions of the court order. The assessor suggested that Mr A might also like somewhere to talk about his feelings and about things that bother him. Over the treatment period of 12 months the weekly sessions developed a pattern. Mr A arrived on time and was always very angry. The first 15–20 minutes involved him aggressively complaining about having to come to the session. He berated the therapist for 'making' him be there and all the other people around him for their intrusions into his life. He shouted and swore, and always refused offers to sit down. He would point at the therapist and shout, 'you're a fucking waste of space, you are', and 'this place is fucking rubbish'. Interestingly, the second half of the sessions were more constructive and there was a marked shift when he started to talk about how the week had been, what had happened at work, etc. However, Mr A remained standing throughout the session.

As the months went on he moved closer and closer to the door, eventually just stepping into the room at the start of the session, shutting the door and then standing without taking his hand off the door handle for almost the whole session. This developed into him slowly turning the door handle as the session progressed, meaning that by the end of the session the handle was fully down and the door ajar. The therapist tried in vain to get Mr A to sit and move away from the door and interpreted his actions in various ways; concerns about safety, not wanting to get too close, getting ready to leave. The therapist tried to engage Mr A in considering what could be achieved, given the limitations of time, and how he got to be in this situation. This process had an impact on the patient's account of his offences. He slowly changed his story so that it became a much more accurate version of what had actually happened. Mr A had developed defences that were rigid and that protected him from his thoughts and feelings. The therapist came to understand Mr A's inner world and found himself confronted with a man struggling with internal and external boundaries. The fantasy of the abandoning mother who continues to live close by but is out of reach, coupled with Mr A's need to hold onto and control the very 'frame' of the treatment were both powerful metaphors of absence and presence, containment and abandonment. Mr A's controlling of the physical boundary of the space was remarkable in that the therapist was able to withstand the angry onslaughts that preceded the emergence of the calmer, less autistic and less disabled man.

There are many areas that have not been discussed in detail here that possibly all of these cases touch on, such as paraphilias and homosexuality, the damage done by abandonment, sexual abuse and the experiences each of these men have in their daily lives.

CONCLUSION

No topic is taboo in the consulting room, but the questions or ideas that a patient is struggling with can elicit complex counter-transference reactions. For Cox (1978) the:

> ...boundary delineation must be established before it is possible to be aware that a boundary has been crossed. (p.238)

Cox points 'to the creative potential of using the boundary of self and others as a "zone" for risk-taking and growth'. However, with patients who are, at best, confused about boundaries this can be a very tall order.

There are inherent difficulties and challenges in assessing and/or treating some patients with learning disabilities, ASD and mental health problems, especially when they are victims of severe boundary violations. The challenges described above can be better understood when thinking about Ogden's (1989) developmental framework of three different modes of generating experience: the paranoid-schizoid, the depressive and the autistic-contiguous. The last one is of most interest in the work described, as it is the most primitive and emerges from an early development of a sense of boundary between self and other at the surface of the skin. Ogden (2008) describes the autistic-contiguous mode of experience as referring:

> ...to the most primitive, healthy psychic organisation. It involves a sensation dominated way of organising experience. (p.224)

Pathological autism can emerge as a result of a combination of constitutional and environmental factors. In an infant or young child an inability to cope with unpredictable external stimuli may lead them to withdraw into a solipsistic and lifeless inner world that is governed by autistic traits. For the patients discussed above this is certainly a feature of their lived experiences.

People who have experienced and lived in the abusive regimes mentioned at the start of the chapter need an opportunity to gain their self-esteem and sense of identity within a therapeutic relationship in order to begin to build a sense of worth, a core part of being able to keep themselves safe in the future. This is also true for the men in the case studies; they too need time and space with a therapist who is not going to react punitively to 'challenging behaviours' and ruptures at the boundary, but is someone who will take the time to explore the experience of being together in the room and focus on the potential for change, as well as how hard it might be to achieve it.

REFERENCES

Alvarez, A. (1992) *Live Company*. London: Routledge.

BBC (2011) 'Four arrests after patient abuse caught on film.' BBC, 1 June 2011. Available at www.bbc.co.uk/news/uk-13548222, accessed on 1 March 2012.

Campbell, D. (1989) 'A psychoanalytic contribution to understanding delinquents at school.' *Journal of Educational Therapy 2*, 4, 50–65.

Corbett, A. (2009) 'Therapy and severe intellectual disability.' In T. Cottis (ed.) *Intellectual Disability, Trauma and Disability*. London: Routledge.

Cox, M. (1978) *Structuring the therapeutic process: Compromise with chaos*. London: Jessica Kingsley Publishers.

Curen, R. (2009) 'Can they see in the door: Assessment and treatment of learning disabled sex offenders.' In T. Cottis (ed.) *Intellectual Disability, Trauma and Disability*. London: Routledge.

EHRC (2011) *Hidden in plain sight: Inquiry into disability-related harassment*. Report by the Equality and Human Rights Commission, August 2011. Available at www.equalityhumanrights.com/uploaded_files/disabilityfi/ehrc_hidden_in_plain_sight_3.pdf, accessed on 1 March 2012.

Glasser, D. (1996) 'Child abuse and neglect and the brain: A review.' *Journal of Child Psychology 41*, 1, 97–116.

Meltzer, D. (1994) 'Impressions concerning adolescent confusional states.' In A. Hahn (ed.) *Sincerity and other works: collected papers of Donald Meltzer*. London: Karnac.

NCCL (1951) *50,000 outside the law: an examination of those certified as mental defectives*. London: The National Council for Civil Liberties.

Ogden, T.H. (1989) *The primitive edge of experience*. Northvale, NJ: Jason Aronson.

Ogden, T. (2008) 'Working analytically with autistic-contiguous aspects of experience.' In K. Barrows (ed.) *Autism in Childhood and Autistic Features in Adults: A Psychoanalytic Perspective*. London: Karnac.

Pring, J. (2011) *Longcare Survivors: the biography of a care scandal*. York: Disability News Service.

Sinason, V. (1989) 'Uncovering and responding to sexual abuse in psychotherapeutic settings.' In H. Brown and A. Craft (eds) *Thinking the Unthinkable: Papers on Sexual Abuse and People with Learning Difficulties*. London: FPA Education Unit.

Sinason, V. (1992) *Mental Handicap and the Human Condition: New approaches from the Tavistock*. London: Free Association Books.

Sinason, V. (1994) 'The treatment of people with learning disabilities who have been abused.' In J. Harris and A. Craft (eds) *People With Learning Disabilities at Risk of Physical or Sexual Abuse*. Kidderminster: British Institute of Learning Disabilities.

Chapter 19

'DANGEROUS LIAISONS': CLOSE ENCOUNTERS OF THE UNBOUNDARIED KIND

Christopher Scanlon and John Adlam[1]

Keep your friends close, and your enemies closer.

Sun-tzu, *Chinese military strategist* (c.400 BC)

Overview

Front-line workers in secure forensic mental health settings, particularly nursing staff, are expected, on behalf of us all, to keep watch over their patients. They must closely observe and assess the movements and behavioural patterns of their patients, whilst themselves being subject to close scrutiny, inspection and surveillance from the wider system of care. Everyone is watching everyone and everyone is on their guard, both dependent upon and under threat from the treatment they receive from their watchers. There is nowhere for either group to hide to escape the scrutiny of the other. In this chapter we reflect upon the boundariless world of what we call the perverse panopticon and we explore the 'dangerous liaisons' that are played out between these would-be watchers and their hyper-vigilant charges. We also discuss the ever-present dynamics of shame and shaming: the illicit excitements that become invested in 'the gaze' and in the reciprocal roles of voyeur and exhibitionist as they pass between the watcher(s) and the watched.

---

1   This chapter is based on and adapted from a longer paper published in *Organisational and Social Dynamics 11*, 2, 175–195, under the title 'Who watches the watchers? Observing the dangerous liaisons between forensic patients and their carers in the *perverse panopticon*.'

INTRODUCTION

In the late 1780s Jeremy Bentham, the British Utilitarian philosopher, proposed the implementation of the 'panopticon' for use in the correction of deviance, antisocial behaviour and criminality. The panopticon (Figure 19.1) was a design for a form of 'correctional facility' in which the living quarters of the inmates would be sufficiently transparent that the 'deviants' could be viewed from all angles at any time by remotely located, unseen attendants, without them being able to tell whether or not they were being watched. Bentham's notion was that the panopticon, as a kind of therapeutic milieu, would give rise to states of mind within which the unseen shaming scrutiny of others would induce pro-social attitudes that would in turn force the offender to reflect upon his/her behaviour and so come to appreciate the error of his/her ways. Bentham himself described the Panopticon as 'a new mode of obtaining power of mind over mind, in a quantity hitherto without example' (Bentham, cited in Bosovic 1995, p.31).

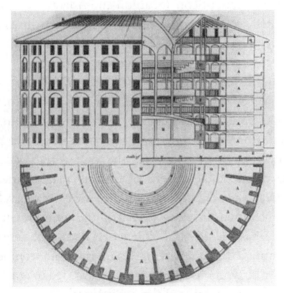

Figure 19.1 Drawing of Bentham's panopticon
(see http://en.wikipedia.org/wiki/Panopticon for discussion)

In his use of the concept Foucault (1975) widened out the panopticon to describe and critique wider social implications in the modern age for state regulation and surveillance as means of governing, through controlling, the wider citizenry. He used the image of 'plague' as a metaphor for the need of the state to exercise this control in order to protect the population from contamination (we have explored elsewhere [Scanlon and Adlam 2009a] how similar ideas are evoked and explored by Albert Camus [1947] in his allegorical novel *La Peste*). Drawing comparisons with the potential for a bodily contamination or infection through leprosy, Foucault suggested that madness and criminality too brought with them a fear of contagion and pointed to a deep-seated social fear that deviance and indiscipline was 'catching', bringing forth a societal response which required that *the mad, the bad and the sad*, like the lepers, needed to be removed from society and confined, under surveillance, until they were seen to be no longer so disturbing.

In our clinical practice we have observed an analogous fear in staff working in secure psychiatric settings in which there is a curious perversion of the dynamic of the panopticon brought about, in part at least, by the contemporary architecture and design of such secure accommodation (Freestone 2005) and in part by the proximity of staff and patients. Nursing stations that were set up to enable nurses to observe patients have also become goldfish bowls within which nursing staff can be constantly observed and scrutinised by the patients. This reciprocal process of observation and scrutiny in itself creates what we have called a 'perverse panopticon' (Scanlon and Adlam 2011) in which all are observed and related to by all – through conscious and intentional scrutiny, as well as the more primitive forms of unconscious communication rooted in processes of projective and introjective identification.

Rather than socialising, the perverse panopticon provides a context within which pro-social forces can be corrupted and staff, as the arbiters of some of these would-be pro-social forces, can become 'contaminated'. In their contaminated states of mind, they then present a clear and present danger to those who they watch over. As was the case with Foucault's historical lazar-houses and the fictional citizens of Camus' plague-stricken town, the anxiety of the perverse panopticon gives rise to a very real psychosomatic fear of relationally transmitted dis-eases as well as the omnipresent threat that it might manifest itself as real physical violence. It is as if the very atmosphere of the ward is contaminated by a terrifying yet invisible environmental pollution which cannot easily be symbolised, nor can it be avoided or ignored – regardless of whether or not one is a wearer of the 'white coat'.

In the forensic treatment setting each party is watching the other for any sign of the aggression, violence or seduction which might put them in harm's way. There is a persistent threat to psychic survival faced both by the workers and the patients inhabiting these boundariless universes where the intrusiveness of looking and being looked at is everywhere. In this perverse and 'unboundaried' environment the very real dangerousness of the patient mirrors the ways in which they experience themselves as endangered by the boundariless and perverted advances of the would-be helper and vice versa. In these settings there is nowhere for either sub-group to hide: no-one will spare your blushes, everyone will hear you scream and even 'angels fear to tread' (Dartington 1994).

ORGANISATIONAL STRUCTURES AND INSTITUTIONALISED VIOLENCE

Quis custodiet ipsos custodes?

Juvenal, *Satires* 6: 346–48

A substantial literature explores the existence and persistence of 'brutal cultures' in forensic settings (e.g. Adlam and Scanlon 2005; Adlam *et al.* 2012; Campling, Aiyegbusi and Clarke-Moore 2009; Davies and Farquharson 2004; Carlyle and Evans 2005; Gilligan 1996; Gordon and Kirtchuk 2008; Hinshelwood 2002; Hopper 2003, 2012; Norton and Dolan 1995; Scanlon and Adlam 2009a). In these brutal cultures, someone is always pushing someone around, and sometimes it appears that everyone is pushing everyone around. The unbearably shaming and unthinkable grief, or more accurately, the conscious and unconsciously contemptuous grievance that attempts to defend against it, is the unbounded, relationally transmitted dis-ease which contaminates the dangerously intimate liaisons within which all parties must work, and live, cheek by jowl, in these enforced, hostile and polluted, exhibitionistic-voyeuristic interdependencies.

Here we are also reminded that Juvenal's poetic question, posed at the beginning of this section, was asked in relation to the imagined impossibility of ensuring that those men whose duty it was to watch over the women of the harem would not be corrupted by, or corrupting in, these duties. The uncorrupted quarantining of a harem presents us, and Juvenal, with the fantasy of being able to achieve a near-impossible task and in the context in which we use it here, we suggest that the forensic system may be understood as re-presenting a contemporary example of exactly such a phenomenon. There is, to be sure, a system boundary, designed, like the boundary of the harem, so that no one may escape, but, unlike the harem, it is designed (albeit imperfectly) so that some of its inmates may eventually pass back out into the boundaried world outside. However, within the system boundary, there is felt to be no limit to the proliferation of perverse enactment.

We would like to invite discussion of one contemporary example of the 'institutionalised' fear of metaphorical corruption in the perverse panopticon. This is the introduction of 'policies' which require front-line workers to wear small bottles of disinfectant on the 'utility belt', which also contains their keys, badges, personal alarms and other powerfully symbolic 'paraphernalia of their office'. This policy was introduced in the winter of 2009 when there was a very real concern about an influenza pandemic in the UK: however, despite the fact that there were few reported cases in psychiatric hospitals and that the public health risk abated, nurses are still required to carry and to use their disinfectant bottles. Could this now institutionalised policy be understood as also a manifestation of a modern social defence (Menzies 1959) that is being deployed to defend against the kind of fear of psychological contamination that we have observed above?

Evidence for this hypothesis might be cited in relation to the operationalisation of the policy. If the policy really was to reduce the risk of cross-infection (rather than an infection of *crossness*), then surely it would have made sense to also offer these disinfectant bottles to the patients, as they are the ones living together 24 hours a day. But the patients are not offered disinfectant bottles and this begs the question who is protecting whom from what? What is a psychotic patient to make of nurses 'disinfecting themselves' following contact with them? Who do they imagine might infect whom, and with what? Could it also be that this practice persists, despite the minuscule risk of actual cross-infection, not only as a social defence against anxiety but also as a concrete manifestation of an institutionalised violence which serves to keep the mentally disordered offender patients firmly in their proper, patronised, disempowered and humiliated place?

The patient in the secure unit has to endure on a daily basis, at great cost to their health, the humiliating experience of their relative poverty and disadvantage (and infectiousness) as they watch, with understandable hatred and envy, those who watch them as they come and go to and from their own homes. For their part, their watchers experience a parallel potential for humiliation and cost to their health and well-being when their needs are denied by those relatively advantaged others who 'manage' and 'direct' them in their work. To give an example of an act of institutional violence done to all, from our own recent experience: a nursing team on a 'Psychiatric Intensive Care Unit' (PICU) were reminded of their worth when, due to economic pressures, their only seclusion room – a powerful tool in their armoury for managing frequent patient violence – was 'decommissioned' so that it could be turned into another bedroom, resulting in an increase in patient numbers and a corresponding increase in the threat of humiliating violence from the patients as well as simultaneously decreasing the staff's capacity to manage it.

This polluted atmosphere of the potential perverse panopticon links also to one part of what Zizek (2008) calls 'objective violence', the invisible background out of which an individual act of subjective violence emerges. For Zizek, this objective, structural violence is always also manifested symbolically, such as the perversion of language which we observe in the day-to-day work in the forensic setting. The contemptuous familiarity contained in terms such as 'attention-seeking', 'manipulative' or 'behavioural', which attribute a rational intentionality to patients' acting-out of their unbearable and unthinkable experience of disempowerment and humiliation, are examples of how such symbolic violence is 'done unto' the patient population (Adlam *et al.* 2012: Aiyegbusi and Clarke-Moore 2009; Chapman 1983; Kelly and May 1982; Norton and Dolan 1995; Scanlon and Adlam 2009b). Likewise, the persistent spoken and unspoken threat – 'We'll have your PIN for this' – reminds us that such symbolic violence can be directed at relatively disadvantaged staff too. They too can be stripped of their identities in a moment. The unthinking wearing of a disinfectant bottle also might be taken as a powerful symbolic communication to remind the mentally disordered offender, and the forensic workers, both of the reality of the patients' guilt and shame and the 'dirtiness' of his/her deeds; as might the thoughtless risk to the health and safety of all caused by the 'decommissioning' of a seclusion room which clearly points to a cynical economic ruthlessness by those who are then experienced as 'knowing the price of everything and the value of nothing' (Oscar Wilde).

WORKING WITH MENTALLY DISORDERED OFFENDERS IN A CULTURE OF SURVEILLANCE

For now we see through a glass, darkly; but then face to face.

Corinthians, 1: 13

Foucault (1975) commented that the major effect of Bentham's pro-social panopticon was 'to induce in the inmate a state of conscious and permanent visibility that assures the automatic functioning of power' (p.201). For this to be effective, the inmate must know that he is being observed; at the same time it must not matter whether he is actually the object of scrutiny at any given moment. The unmeasurable and unknowable possibility of being observed is enough to ensure security and compliance and so enable a mending of deviant ways. The panopticon, Foucault points out, separates two experiences that are normally linked: that of seeing and being seen: 'in the peripheric ring, one is totally seen, without ever seeing; in the central tower, one sees everything without ever being seen' (1975, p.202). Bentham's panopticon also problematically relies upon an assumption of the 'good intentions' of those who construct the prison and define the boundaries and rules of engagement: however, in the perverse panopticon, neither of these conditions can be guaranteed. In the perverse panopticon the looker and the looked at, the voyeur and the exhibitionist, are both perfectly catered for only if they are clearly differentiated and each is in their proper respective place and in a familiar, ego-syntonic state of mind. They are utterly frustrated if they are undifferentiated, 'in the other's place' or in an unfamiliar or ego-dystonic state of mind.

Now, we know from experience that the 'close observation' of disturbed patients on contemporary inpatient units is no guarantee that the object of this 'therapeutic surveillance' will 'mend' his or her ways. On the contrary, this technique often creates a highly charged and uniquely perverse game of hide-and-seek, which even at its most benign is an expression of the exhibitionist–voyeur dynamic highlighted above that can be exhausting for both parties. At its most malign, it can provide an invitation, from one or other party, to reinforce and to gratify more toxic, highly sexualised sado-masochistic engagements that have an inherent potential to corrupt and debase (Jukes 1997; Motz 2008; Welldon 1996). During the more physical of these encounters nursing staff (men and women) can be sadistically attacked by patients (women and men) who unconsciously parallel and re-create their own violent, sadistic and often highly sexualised patterns of offending in the here-and-now of their encounters in the ward (Norton and Dolan 1995; Shine and Morris 2000).

At other times this perverse desire for bodily contact inverts as well as perverts the victim–perpetrator dynamics, as nurses are recruited by the masochistic part of patients' minds 'to put them down'. This often unconsciously sexualised problem is made all the more acute when the seclusion room has been made unavailable, requiring that patients, in these highly charged, 'post-coital' states of minds, have to be taken back to their own bedroom to be settled. Although we think we know some of this, under extreme provocation, and mired in the blood and spittle of the highly charged perverse panopticon, there is little space to think and so little opportunity to learn very much from this experience. Indeed, in these highly charged and highly traumatised environments there is often little incentive to come together to learn from experience when this would involve having to consider the interpersonal and psychosocial meaning of these often violent and highly sexualised interactions that cast forensic workers in roles that are ego-dystonic and very disturbing (Gabbard and Wilkinson 1994; Gordon and Kirtchuk 2008; Hopper 2003, 2012; Scanlon and Adlam 2009a, 2012).

Under the conditions of the 'perverse panopticon' it is therefore often the nursing staff who are forced to take up the position formerly occupied, in Bentham's imagination, by the miscreant: that of being the focus of scrutiny and challenge. Except that, rather than being subject to pro-social forces from the healthy parts of the patients' and the systems' minds, they feel themselves to be constantly watched, not only by the patients, but also by their friends in the 'management'. As we have described elsewhere (Scanlon and Adlam 2009a) nurses often describe their experience as if they were combatants on a battlefield upon which there is both hostile and friendly fire.

In the clinical arena some of the 'hostile fire' comes in the form of symbolic and concrete appeasement, seduction and grooming of staff by patients, and of patients by staff, which seem ostensibly 'friendly', making matters even more confusing. In the organisational context the 'friendly fire' takes the form of ever greater scrutiny from ever more demanding managerial and institutional systems of governance. These demands typically involve the insatiable need to do more for less (as in the example of the decommissioned seclusion room). This is coupled with and operationalised through the widespread implementation of technologies in which interventions can be monitored by remote and faceless technicians who proceed on the basis that if it is not recorded on the electronic systems then it did not happen. The 'Wizard of Oz' behind the technological screens of remote surveillance is often part of an incontinent management culture experienced as pouncing on any mistake and subjecting its maker to the 'third degree' in an increasingly structurally violent culture of inquiry, inspection, blame and recrimination (Cooper and Lousada 2005; Rustin 2004a, 2004b) within which the usual ethic that presumes innocence until proven guilty is inverted and perverted as staff come to experience the default position as guilty until proven innocent.

Whether any of these measures have a remedial effect on bad practice, we may doubt; but in our experience they do induce a sense of fear and loathing of the 'Wizard' in many able and experienced practitioners. The effect is to move away from greater relational security, reflective practice and team development (Pfäfflin and Adshead 2004; Scanlon 2012; Scanlon and Adlam 2012) and inevitably towards an anxious attachment rooted in a preoccupation with personal survival, physical security and manifested in a panoply of offensive and defensive practice measures (Adlam *et al.* 2012; Aiyegbusi and Clarke-Moore 2009; Gordon and Kirtchuk 2008; Scanlon and Adlam 2009a, 2011b). Whether the focus is on hostile or on friendly fire, our observation is that the anxiety generated by these skirmishes increases the likelihood that staff and patients alike will be locked together into the potentially boundariless contaminations of the perverse panopticon.

It is often observed that the ward staff who are most often charged with taking up an exposed position in order 'to observe' patients are often the most junior or least-well-trained staff. As well as watching out for signs of danger, their job is also essentially to watch over, protect, look after and care about the objects of their gaze. To gaze at another is an intimate and engaging transaction: an invitation, either to avert your gaze or to look back, to reciprocate. Furthermore, the patients are not merely the passive recipients of this scrutiny. They too are gazing into the others' eyes, watching very carefully, often to identify a perceived weakness: for opportunity to offend, or to give offence. Sometimes they are looking out for ordinary human intimacy; and at other times the need or wish is to seduce, reduce or debase. This is a very intimate form of confinement which brings with it all manner of intimate desires as well as a full range of weaponry to fight against it.

The nursing staff in these settings find themselves unwittingly the very embodiment of the dream that Bentham had for his prospective prisoners, which Foucault summarises as 'the principle that power should be visible and unverifiable' (1975, p.201): they are thus controlled into a position where, caught between the ever-present scrutinies of both the patients and 'the establishment', they end up exercising the persecutory surveillance upon themselves. Watchers are not entirely dispensed with, of course, but neither are they any longer strictly necessary. The simple possibility of being 'caught out' in some way, whether by patients, supervisors, managers or so-called whistle-blowers, suffices.

CONCLUSION: THE CONCEPT OF BOUNDARIES IN A FREE-FIRE ZONE

The intersection between staff and patients in the conditions of the perverse panopticon comes to be experienced on all sides as a kind of 'no-man's land' in which workers and patients face each other and throughout which fearful communications of various sorts are being constantly projected. In this chapter we are emphasising the visual nature and domain of this barrage of projectiles. The forensic setting, understood in these terms, can then be compared to a boundariless 'combat zone' where watching and being watched are the weapons of war and the projectiles are missiles of shame and humiliation and of grievance born of an incapacity to grieve. The forensic inpatient nurse and the forensic patients are cooped up together in a most hazardous double jeopardy. Within the system boundary, as with the guards and the harem of Juvenal's satire, there is the too-intimate enforced proximity and dis-ease of a closed community where sex and violence is on everyone's mind but no one can speak of it; across the system boundary, there is the painful awareness of the hostility and equally the prurience of the outside world, public opinion, government policy and homeland security that seeks to ensure that this disease is effectively quarantined.

The watchers and the watched are pinned down by each other's scrutiny, undifferentiated and indistinguishable from each other in their reciprocal roles. There is a precarious co-existence, to be sure, but this is sustained in or despite the shared knowledge that, at any moment, a colleague or a fellow patient may put a foot momentarily wrong and be picked off by enemy snipers – or bureaucratic decisions made far away from the battlefield. As Gilligan (1996) observed, in such settings and under these circumstances violence, and the fear of violence, has indeed become a potentially deadly 'epidemic'. Insofar as this reciprocal violence is expressed visually, in the sadism of the voyeur and the masochism of the exhibitionist, the risk of contagion and the impossibility of quarantine is felt to be greater, the greater the visibility and equivalent lack of privacy of the setting. In this context Juvenal's age-old philosophical question about 'who watches the watchmen' has perhaps never been more relevant and immediate.

REFERENCES

Adlam, J., Aiyegbusi, A., Kleinot, P., Motz, A. and Scanlon, C. (2012) (eds) *The Therapeutic Milieu Under Fire: Security and Insecurity in Forensic Mental Health*. London: Jessica Kingsley Publishers.

Adlam, J. and Scanlon, C. (2005) 'Personality disorder and homelessness: membership and "unhoused minds" in forensic settings.' *Group Analysis 38*, 3, 452–466. Special Issue – Group Analysis in Forensic Settings.

Aiyegbusi, A. and Clarke-Moore, J. (2009) (eds) *Relationships with Offenders: An Introduction to the Psychodynamics of Forensic Mental Health Nursing*. London: Jessica Kingsley Publishers.

Bentham, J. (1995) *Panopticon (Preface)*. In M. Bozovic (ed.) *The Panopticon Writings*. London: Verso.

Campling, P., Davies, S. and Farquharson, G. (2004) (eds) *From Toxic Institutions to Therapeutic Environments: Residential Settings in Mental Health Services*. London: Gaskell.

Camus, A. (1947) *La Peste (The Plague)*. New York: Vintage Books.

Carlyle, J. and Evans, C. (2005) 'Containing containers: attention to the "innerface" and "outerface" of groups in secure institutions.' *Group Analysis 38*, 3, 395–408.

Chapman, G.E. (1983) 'Ritual and rational action in hospitals.' *Journal of Advanced Nursing 8*, 13–20.

Cooper, A. and Lousada, J. (2005) *Borderline Welfare: Feeling and Fear of Feeling in Modern Welfare*. London: Karnac.

Dartington, A. (1994) 'Where Angels Fear to Tread: Idealism, despondency and opportunities for thought in hospital nursing.' In A. Obholzer and V. Zagier Roberts (eds) *The Unconscious at Work: Individual and Organizational Stress in the Human Services*. London: Routledge.

Foucault, M. (1975) *Discipline and Punish: The Birth of the Prison*. New York: Vintage Books.

Freestone, M. (2005) 'Overview of an ethnographic study of the UK DSPD pilot units.' *Therapeutic Communities 26*, 4, 449–464.

Gabbard, G.O. and Wilkinson, S.M. (1994) 'Holding, Containment and Thinking One's Own Thoughts.' In G.O. Gabbard and S.M. Wilkinson (eds) *Management of Counter-transference with Borderline Patients*. Washington, DC: American Psychiatric Press.

Gilligan, J. (1996) *Violence: Reflections on our Deadliest Epidemic*. London: Jessica Kingsley Publishers.

Gordon, J. and Kirtchuk, G. (2008) *Psychic Assaults and Frightened Clinicians: Countertransference in Forensic Settings*. London: Karnac.

Hinshelwood, R.D. (2002) 'Abusive help – Helping Abuse: The Psychodynamic Impact of Severe Personality Disorder on Caring Institutions.' *Criminal Behaviour and Mental Health 12*, 2, 20–31.

Hopper, E. (2003) *Traumatic Experience in the Unconscious Life of Groups: The Fourth Basic Assumption: Incohesion: Aggregation/Massification or (ba) I:A/M*. London: Jessica Kingsley Publishers.

Hopper, E. (2012) *Trauma In Organisations*. London: Karnac.

Jukes, A. (1997) *Why Men Hate Women*. London: Free Associations.

Kelly, M.P. and May, D. (1982) 'Good and bad patients: A review of the literature and a theoretical critique.' *Journal of Advanced Nursing 7*, 147–156.

Menzies, I.E.P. (1959) 'The functioning of social systems as a defence against anxiety – a report on a study of the nursing service within a general hospital.' *Human Relations 13*, 95–121.

Motz, A. (2008) *The Psychology of Female Violence: Crimes Against the Body* (2nd edn). London: Routledge.

Norton, K. and Dolan, B. (1995) 'Acting out and the institutional response.' *Journal of Forensic Psychiatry 6*, 317–332.

Pfäfflin, F. and Adshead, G. (2004) (eds) *A Matter of Security: The Application of Attachment Theory to Forensic Psychiatry and Psychotherapy*. London: Jessica Kingsley Publishers.

Rustin, M.J. (2004a) 'Re-thinking Audit and Inspection.' *Soundings 64*, 86–107.

Rustin, M.J. (2004b) 'Learning from the Victoria Climbié Inquiry.' *Journal of Social Work Practice 18*, 1, 9–18.

Scanlon, C. (2012) 'The Traumatised Organisation-in-the-mind: Creating and maintaining spaces for difficult conversations in difficult places' in J. Adlam, A. Aiyegbusi, P. Kleinot, A. Motz and C. Scanlon (eds). *The Therapeutic Milieu Under Fire: Security and Insecurity in Forensic Mental Health*. London: Jessica Kingsley Publishers.

Scanlon, C. and Adlam, J. (2009a) 'Nursing dangerousness, dangerous nursing and the spaces in between: learning to live with uncertainties.' In A. Aiyegbusi and J. Clarke-Moore (eds) *Relationships with Offenders: An Introduction to the Psychodynamics of Forensic Mental Health Nursing*. London: Jessica Kingsley Publishers.

Scanlon, C. and Adlam, J. (2009b) '"Why do you treat me this way?": reciprocal violence and the mythology of "deliberate self harm".' In A. Motz (ed.) *Managing Self Harm: Psychological Perspectives*. London: Taylor and Francis.

Scanlon, C. and Adlam, J. (2011) '*Who watches the watchers?* Observing the dangerous liaisons between forensic patients and their carers in the *perverse panopticon*'. *Organisational and Social Dynamics 11*, 2, 175–195.

Scanlon, C. and Adlam, J. (2012) 'Disorganised responses to refusal and spoiling in traumatised organisations.' In E. Hopper (ed.) *Trauma in Organisations*. London: Karnac.

Shine, J., and Morris, M. (2000) 'Addressing *criminogenic* needs in a prison therapeutic community.' *Therapeutic Communities 21*, 197–219.

Welldon, E.V. (1996) 'Contrasts in Male and Female Perversions.' In C. Cordess and M. Cox (eds) *Forensic Psychotherapy: Crime, Psychodynamics and the Offender Patient*. London: Jessica Kingsley Publishers.

Zizek, S. (2008) *Violence*. London: Profile Books.

Chapter 20

NEITHER HERE NOR THERE, NOT ONE THING OR ANOTHER: THE USE OF A REFLECTIVE PRACTICE GROUP TO UNDERSTAND THE DISTORTION OF A BOUNDARY

Stephen Mackie

Overview

This is a book about boundaries: what they are, why they are important, how and why they may be attacked, and what occurs when a boundary is broken. The term 'boundary' denotes a structure of some form, with its order, rules and clarity. The aim of the structure is to provide containment. As boundaries separate one time and/or space from another, separation and difference are also acknowledged. Psychically, having our own internal space, our mind, with its own structure and boundaries allows us to be able to think and to have 'minds of our own' and therefore an individual sense of identity.

There are times, however, when boundaries themselves are defensively acted upon and distorted in order to avoid clarity, to avoid the pain of knowing or being known. Mental pain is thus avoided but at the cost of containment.

INTRODUCTION

The term 'boundary' denotes a structure of some form, with its order, rules and clarity. The aim of the structure is to provide containment. As boundaries separate one time and/or space from another, separation and difference are also acknowledged. Psychically, having our own internal space, our mind, with its own structure and boundaries allows us to be able to think and to have 'minds of our own' and therefore an individual sense of identity.

In this chapter I wish to explore one particular example of when the specificity of the boundary in a psychiatric ward staff team appears to be avoided or absent and therefore clarity, including clarity of task and of thought, is seriously affected. Instead of being specific and delineated, the boundary becomes widened and develops into a hidden protective space in itself. The aim of this space is to distort boundaries and structure.

I will use material from a reflective practice group as an example of such a space and of its use by the members who inhabit it. Reflective practice groups provide a window into the culture, dynamics, anxieties and defences of a particular ward, team or unit and so functions as a microcosm of the wider field offering detailed research by its participants of their larger environment. Issues that arise within the ward, team or unit, whether healthy or unhealthy, are often repeated or enacted in a reflective practice group. That is, the pertinent issues of that particular time are brought to the group, hopefully for exploration and understanding. In the reflective practice group I will describe, the group is being used to keep difficult experiences and thoughts at bay. Problems and difficulties were to be kept out of the group, 'out there'.

John Steiner coined the term 'psychic retreat' to denote withdrawn states of mind that provide relative peace and protection from strain when interpersonal contact seems painful and threatening. He believed that 'when transient, such states pose little difficulty and might even be ego-replenishing. However, turning to these retreats habitually and tenaciously can pose a serious challenge to conducting analysis. Meaningful contact with the analyst is experienced as threatening' (Steiner 1993). This position for Steiner is a borderline position used in order to avoid both paranoid and depressive anxieties.

O'Shaughnessy (1992) describes what she calls an enclave: a psychological organisation which deforms an essential feature of psychoanalysis. That is, its openness to possibilities of disturbance and the knowing of new areas.

THE AIMS OF A REFLECTIVE PRACTICE GROUP

Within a psychodynamic frame, the use of individual, team or ward reflective practice is one method of supporting and helping staff tolerate difficult emotions and experiences. The aim is to create a reflective space, whereby an understanding of staff's anxieties, and the source of these anxieties, can be attempted. Our anxiety becomes more tolerable and manageable when it is more understood or, in other words, thought about.

The aim of this form of support is therefore to try to help staff broaden their spectrum of awareness, thinking and feeling in order to allow them to be more free and able to think about their clinical and work issues, how they feel about them and to make decisions based upon that thinking and feeling. Support is therefore obtained through understanding. In the example that I am about to describe, the aims and structures of the reflective practice group were themselves distorted in order to create a space where emotional contact, and therefore understanding, was to be avoided.

Example

I had been asked to facilitate a reflective practice group on a psychiatric rehabilitation ward. I was never able to elicit from the senior nurse managers what they felt the difficulties on the ward were or what they hoped the group would achieve. They had an idea that something was not right but could not clarify precisely what. It felt to me that they were having difficulty attending to something specific. From the beginning, clarity and specifics were either hidden or absent to the point that even agreeing on a start date, the initial group boundary, was difficult. Indeed, there was never a clear boundary to the starting of each group.

Although I facilitated the group on the same day and time, for the first year my weekly arrival on the ward appeared to be an unexpected occurrence for the staff. I felt that I did not really exist for the staff. I would be taken to the nursing station and left there, seen but not really acknowledged, often left in this position for some time feeling irritated, frustrated, unattended to, left in limbo, controlled and powerless. My presence was being turned 'a blind eye to' by the nursing staff. I felt that if I said anything clearly about the situation that I found myself in, it would be heard as a complaint; and although I did wish to complain, I wondered if the team may be, at some level, communicating to me something of their own work experience – that of feeling neglected and angry, disempowered and controlled and lost as to what to do. I felt a subtle pressure and expectation to just 'go through the motions' and collude with a position whereby everything was to be kept unspecified, hazy and 'cloudy'. I should not protest or make any comment but remain in a deeply unsatisfying place. I should not 'rock the boat'.

I found it difficult to attend to and be clear in my own thinking during these groups. I felt that the group made a form of pseudo-contact; events and situations were discussed and talked about, little of which made any real emotional impact on me. There was little actual material that I could use to build thoughts with and I had the sense of not only 'going through the motions' but being expected to just go through the motions with everyone else. Over time I began to despair about the group ever achieving anything of value.

The room we met in had unplastered but painted brick walls, and during groups where I found it particularly difficult to think clearly I would occasionally find myself free associating to this wall; a clear, distinct and concrete boundary, in contrast to my experiences. I recalled that the mortar was not used to bind the bricks together but to keep them apart in order to allow a degree of give in the structure and so avoid catastrophic collapse when the stresses and strains on the structure exceeded its tolerance limit. I recounted that the name of the older material, used before mortar, lime, is derived from the Latin 'limin' meaning threshold, the space one enters when leaving one space and before entering another. The space is neither here nor there, not one place or another. These associations later helped me to construct some ideas, some structured thoughts, about what may be occurring.

In a later meeting the ward staff chose to discuss a particularly difficult patient on their ward who they were struggling to tolerate. He did not engage with them, listen to them or take anything helpful from them. He frustrated and disempowered the staff and they were lost as to what to do with him. He looked down upon their attempts to help him.

Although the stated aim of the ward was that of rehabilitation (whatever that may actually mean in practice) it was clear that their patient could not cope out in the wider community. Out there he felt very small and inadequate. On the ward he turned the tables, putting staff in this position of feeling inadequate and lost whereas he could feel 'big' and powerful. The staff felt powerless because their organisation expected them to 'rehabilitate' this man, move him on to the community, but he would resist all their efforts, as he was frightened. The expectations they felt placed upon them did not meet the reality of the situation they were in. The aims of their ward and the needs of the patient did not seem to match; there was no common sense of task. They therefore had to 'fail'.

They told me that their patient perpetually wandered the corridors of the ward, spending only short amounts of time in any room. It was as if he felt most at ease in not one place or another. As an apparent aside, one nurse then told the others of his method of disciplining his young son when he was naughty, or we could say, did something his parents disapproved of. He told us that at these times he would place his son on the stairs, half-way up and half-way down; not one place or another. His anecdote brought to my mind my own experiences while left in the nursing station: put half-way up the stairs, powerless and isolated, a place where nothing happens.

This, for the patient, was a safe place away from feeling small, hopeless and depressed on the downstairs floor, the 'grounded' one where he had painful insight into the reality of his predicament and felt scared and powerless. The alternative to this place was a manic flight to the upstairs; a more paranoid place of being high, superior, looking down contemptuously upon normal human pain, worries, anxieties, vulnerabilities and needs. Up here he would be threatening and controlling, violent if necessary in order to control others in order to project his feelings of being small and inadequate into the staff.

I felt this may also have reflected the staff's experience, that they felt helpless in their attempts to rehabilitate or change his behaviour and therefore felt that they had failed. One defence against this guilt and despair would be a flight from it to a more paranoid position, above failure. I used my associations about the brick wall and the 'limin' and wondered if an enclave would provide relief from both these positions. Steiner writes that the retreat 'then serves as an area of mind where reality does not have to be faced, where phantasy and omnipotence can exist unchecked and where anything is possible' (Steiner 1993, p.1). He believed that it is this feature that makes the retreat so attractive, that people retreat behind 'a powerful system of defences which serve as a protective armour or hiding place' (Steiner 1993, p.3).

The staff actually wanted to get rid of their patient and hoped that he would be transferred to another unit or hospital that had 'more experience and skills' as they did not feel that they could meet his needs or give him what he wanted: 'We don't have the resources required to care for him.' They did not have the 'magic cure' that they felt was required and expected of them.

I also felt that the staff wanted to get rid of something else, but this time from within themselves. I felt that they wanted rid of their own awareness and capacities to think. To think would mean making contact with what they felt – in this case, painful feelings of helplessness, vulnerability, failure and powerlessness. There were limitations to what they could do and there was no magic. Their retreat, when functioning well, allowed them to maintain omnipotent phantasies that they could get rid of all problems.

I told the group that they had found it difficult to let me know about their complaint, their pain and worries, as they had concerns as to whether I would acknowledge their experiences or judge and criticise them instead. That perhaps they also had difficulties doing the same with themselves, acknowledging their true feelings by placing themselves half-way up and half-way down the stairs.

One nurse responded to my intervention by complaining that they were not given adequate resources to do their job. She continued that there had recently been an incident on the ward where a nurse had felt seriously threatened by a patient and very few nursing colleagues from other wards responded to the alarm when activated. When she and some of her colleagues approached other wards to complain about this they were told that the alarms either did not work properly or, on some wards, had been turned off due to the high number of false alarms. This nurse was in touch with her fears for her own safety and complained that when she brought her professional concerns to her management she felt accused of not being 'up to the job'. As a result she would find herself questioning (that is undermining) her capacities as a nurse. As she made contact with herself and her true feelings she realised that she was extremely frustrated and angry. She complained that her pain, and her fears, had not been acknowledged. At the end of the group she complained of having developed a headache. By having the courage to emerge from the retreat and make true contact with herself and her feelings she now felt physical pain. I felt this to be both an acknowledgement of the painful position she found herself in and the result of an internalised attack as retaliation for leaving the retreat. Being clear, hurt.

I suggested to the group that there was a pressure to switch off their own receiving equipment – their common sense – as their alarm was so frequent and overwhelming. After all, they were saying, everyone else is doing so. They had to put on their psychological, but distancing, armour and performed their work in a mechanical manner, turning a 'blind eye' not only to what disturbed them in reality but also to their own feelings and concerns about their own and their patient's predicament. This required a disengagement from their feelings, their work, their patients and the organisation around them. They felt their complaint, their pain, had to be kept hidden.

Once I had made it clear to the nurses that I was able to acknowledge their pain they became able to tell me of a litany of serious assaults that had been occurring, all frightening and never before brought out into the open in the group. I was shocked and surprised by the degree of assault and violence that had been occurring and kept hidden and, as listener, felt rather assaulted myself. They had a complaint that 'no one wanted to know' about their experiences but also did not want anyone to know as this might expose their hidden enclave. The view that 'no one wants to know' also applied to themselves.

The staff seemed in two minds: they valued me as someone who may benevolently 'see' and acknowledge them and their experiences, but also, simultaneously, wanted rid of me as a potential source of knowing (in the transference, the 'patient' that they could not control and wanted rid of). There was the wish to think, to make contact with themselves, alongside the wish to get rid of their thinking. Bion (1962) thought contact, both physical and emotional, could be thought of as a process of containment. To think would bring them into painful contact with their own feelings of loss, including loss of their own idealisation of what could be achieved and what they should be capable of (a perfect cure and a perfect clinician). 'Some complain about their predicament, others however, accept the situation with resignation and relief and, at times, defiance or triumph so that it is the analyst who has to carry the despair associated with the failure to make contact' (Steiner 1993, p.2).

THE SUPEREGO

To attempt to understand some of the reasons why this retreat or enclave may be resorted to it is useful to return to Freud. Freud (1923) described an agency in our minds that he called the superego. This is an agency that oversees and monitors the ego, that part of the mind that is in contact with reality. The superego sees conscience, self-observation and the formation of ideals as its function. It can vary in its harshness, and omnipotently looks down on need or dependency as these do not conform to its demands for the 'ideal', or the perfect. This omnipotent state of affairs is based more upon surveillance, obedience and persecution than on personal freedom to take responsibility. It is freedom and therefore life itself that is to be controlled.

When under pressure, having limited resources and under high performance expectations, organisations such as the NHS, like individual human beings, can become dominated by superego functioning – demanding efficiency, perfection and smooth running, a goal only achievable if everyone is the same, acts the same and thinks the same. Anything that interferes with this demand is to be either controlled, or if control is not possible, got rid of. Need is seen as a weakness as it implies dependency, and therefore vulnerability and pain, which challenges this 'ideal' as in an ideal world there would be no pain. Therefore patients and staff – if viewed as having concerns, anxieties, needs for anything such as leadership, support, concern for their well-being – are to be monitored, controlled or got rid of.

This kind of system, with its processes, monitoring and targets, can set increasingly unrealistic expectations on people. Under the stress of constant change and uncertainty, new models and programmes are created and then re-created when they do not achieve the anticipated miracle, as 'care' is seen as not good enough and is replaced with 'cure'. Concepts such as empathy and common sense, aspects pertaining to our humanity, are devalued and looked down upon.

The two aims, control or care, become increasingly incompatible and at times appear to have little in common. There becomes no sense of a common, shared goal, no 'common sense'. This can leave staff feeling despairing, hopeless and powerless. The option staff then have is to either identify with 'the aggressor', looking down on need, dependency and pain, or, alternatively, be in a low position, despairing, feeling guilty for 'failing' in some way and feeling looked down upon. Neither of these options is particularly palatable. The alternative to these two positions is to create, and enter, the retreat, initially as a temporary measure, although after a time the risk is of becoming stuck.

In my example, the nurses identified three positions that their patient could be in as, I think, indicating the same options for themselves:

1. Upstairs, embracing omnipotent structures in the paranoid schizoid position (Klein 1946) where an aloof, high position is occupied in order to avoid normal human feelings and experiences, including helplessness, need, pain and human limitation. It is a 'hard' position, above real humanity. Need is to be denied and magically done away with. Activity becomes cold and routine, ticking boxes and following 'procedures' in an unthinking manner. Everyone is to be the same, act the same and think the same. Any signs of real need are looked down upon by a critical eye, controlled and attacked, seen as 'soft' or weak.

2. Downstairs, in the depressive position (Klein 1935). This is a low place where people can feel powerless, despairing, hopeless and preoccupied by a feeling of having insufficient resources. Staff in the downstairs position fear being attacked by accusations of 'weakness' or 'not being up to the job' (whatever that may be). Occupying this position allows us to be in touch with our true feelings, but we are therefore confronted with the pain of our limitations. This is a painful position but is the position that carries the hope of recovery if the experience can be tolerated, that is, if the pain can be borne. Support, as a resource, is required for this. This position brings with it a personal sense of failure, although it is actually a failure to maintain the omnipotent demands for the ideal.

3. Half-way up and half-way down (not one place or another). An alternative way of coping with this very difficult choice between 'Up' and 'Down' is to remain hidden in a third position, neither one place nor another, not fully seen or recognised, an enclave where no true contact is made, either with their patients, their profession, their organisation or their own feelings and thoughts. The cost of inhabiting this space is that staff become detached: 'The relief provided by the retreat is achieved at the cost of isolation, stagnation and withdrawal' (Steiner 1993). In this position, being clear and specific in our thinking, knowing our true feelings, such as a wish to complain,

cannot be allowed as it is too risky and risks attack if seen. Any signs of life are to be killed off pre-emptively, clarity and specifics got rid of. This position differs from 'upstairs' in that thinking and reality is not completely denied but there is collusion with the upstairs position by using the sensory apparatus of choice – the 'Blind Eye'.

THE EXPERIENCE OF THE FACILITATOR

This is best described by Steiner's (1993) work with individual patients who use this defensive position and I believe the same is experienced by the facilitator of groups of individuals. He states that, 'he can feel to be getting nowhere for long periods and has to struggle with his own propensity both to fit in and collude with the organisation on the one hand and to withdraw into his own defensive retreat on the other. He is often under great pressure, and his frustration may lead him to despair or to mount a usually futile effort to overcome what are perceived as the patient's stubborn defences' (p.13).

CONCLUSION

To be effective in, and to gain satisfaction from, our work and obtain a personal sense of satisfaction and meaning from what we do, we need to feel emotionally involved – with our patients, our work, our profession and ourselves. We need to attempt to understand our own anxieties and difficulties as well as our patients in order to prevent a defensive distancing from our patients, and so from ourselves.

If there is no acknowledgement of need (pain) in ourselves, as in our patients, there can be no movement, no change and we remain stuck in a timeless, lost place half-way up the stairs or half-way down the stairs, unseen and unacknowledged, trying to please everyone. In this place there is little life and little chance of anything of real meaning occurring. What can remain is the hope that patients will somehow change by just our presence – the placebo effect. When inhabiting the retreat the person or group is protected from these anxieties but then has real problems of identity. Clinicians become not one thing or another. They lose their professional identity, their sense of who they are and what their task is.

Acknowledgement of ourselves requires protected space and time where we can attempt to engage with ourselves and our thoughts and feelings, particularly the emotional pain of our human limitation. Pain and humanity go hand in hand – physical pain, the pain of loss, rejection and the pain of guilt.

I believe that omnipotent systems of thinking are resorted to when the pain of limitation, both institutional and human, cannot be borne. The wish is for the pain, the complaint, to disappear, not exist. In reality, pain will not go away; it will express itself despite this denial. When denied this pain, the complaint is more likely to occur in a sudden, shocking physical manner. It becomes both a traumatic assault on an individual's physical and emotional well-being and can be experienced as an assault on the illusions of an omnipotent system.

REFERENCES

Bion, W. (1962) 'A theory of thinking.' *International Journal of Psychoanalysis 43*, 306–310.

Freud, S. (1923) 'The Ego and the Id.' *The Standard Edition of the Complete Psychological Works of Sigmund Freud*. Vol. 19, 3–64.

Klein, M. (1935) 'A Contribution to the psychogenesis of manic-depressive states.' *International Journal of Psychoanalysis 16*, 145–174.

Klein, M. (1946) 'Notes on some schizoid mechanisms.' *International Journal of Psychoanalysis 27*, 99–110.

O'Shaughnessy, E. (1992) 'Enclaves and Excursions.' *International Journal of Psychoanalysis 73*, 603–611.

Steiner, J. (1993) *Psychic Retreats*. New Library of Psychoanalysis Vol. 19. London: Routledge.

Chapter 21

BOUNDARIES AND HOMICIDE

Ronald Doctor and Maggie McAlister

Overview

Homicide is the ultimate boundary violation. The act of murder is a
trauma that defies the boundary of the other, violently attacks the physical
boundary of the individual and involves the destruction of life itself. The
ultimate transgression into the life of the other is to cross a boundary from
which there is no return: the destruction is irreversible and irreparable.
How do we understand such acts? And how as professionals can we be
aware of re-enactments within our therapeutic relationships? This chapter
will look at the psychopathology of homicide and consider how we can
work effectively and safely with the homicidal patient.

THE PSYCHOPATHOLOGY OF HOMICIDE

In psychoanalytic theory, the Oedipus complex has been recognised as the
central conflict in the human psyche – the essential group of conflicting
impulses, phantasies, anxieties and defences. If we consider the Oedipus myth
from the angle of the role played by the gods we can follow this process. The
god Apollo has ordained that Oedipus would kill his father Laius and marry
his mother Jocasta. Laius' only hope was that the baby Oedipus would not
survive. Oedipus was delivered to a shepherd with orders to abandon him on
a mountain, but human compassion, the antidote to cruelty, intervened and
entrusted the child to a Corinthian shepherd. After unknowingly killing his
father and marrying his mother, Oedipus has to root out his father's murderer
and pursued this course with persistent vigour. The tragic revelation of what he
had done led to his plucking out his eyes and his abandonment to cruel exile.

Thus the violence relates to a core phantasy that involves both the primary relationship with the mother and phantasies about the primal scene, that is, the original act which created the individual. The violence has the function of allowing the perpetrator to believe that he can create a space in which he can survive in the face of an object that is experienced as terrifying. Violence is thus a communication about these patients' belief systems about themselves, about their relationships with others and about their origins. The violent act or phantasy tells a story that represents the patient's personal myth of creation and contains both pre-oedipal and distorted oedipal theories. The function of the therapeutic process is to follow the chains of associations as manifested and enacted in the transference and counter-transference, and to reconstruct the narrative of their origins.

Murder occurs concretely only after it has been committed many times previously in daydreams, nightmares and sometimes in unconscious phantasy that has never become conscious. Before the deed, conscious efforts – sometimes unconscious ones too, both sado-masochistic and psychotic – are designed and devoted to keeping the impulse to murder encapsulated to prevent action. In thinking about boundary violations in homicide, one has to first consider the internal boundary violation, which leads to the concrete action of the murder itself. Then a sudden reversal takes place internally that breaks the murderousness loose from its cordoned-off status, and the energies of the individual become devoted to enacting the murderous deed. The death constellation always includes a psychically traumatic and indigestible experience to do with loss and death.

What is needed is a structure or setting that can take the patient to the crossroads of their origins and to explore how, when he is exiled from the family, the family is in turn exiled from the past, the present and, until their tragic relationship is resolved, the future. The analytic work is about discovering, not the trauma of a singular catastrophe that can be overcome and healed, but a trauma that involves the destruction of life itself. This creates a void, an overwhelming emptiness in which the continuity of life and history is so brutally disrupted that the structure of life is forever torqued and transformed. The patient lives in a world where there is only darkness and nothingness, and they fill this hole with sado-masochism and psychosis. (Doctor 2008)

According to Benjamin (1940), in *Theses on the Philosophy of History*, personal narratives can become fragmented, psychotic and appear like a 'pile of debris', which is at times all that may stand out as intelligible in a life story containing abuse, trauma and psychosis. The psychotic experience can become reified and occupy a disproportionately pre-eminent position in a person's autobiography and its translation by acute psychiatry. The patient's version of history can become devalued and the meaning of the story, in their own words rather than in psychiatric translation, is too often disregarded. For them, the relative vividness of the psychotic experience can stand out against a background of impoverishment; it can form a powerful, collective historical continuum that subsumes the individual history. At this point the ability of the individual to maintain a view of himself that is distinct from the image offered to him by the psychotic spectacle begins to fade. The risk for people with psychosis is that the full complexity of their memories of themselves is fractioned and distilled, leaving only the most potent of images to represent them. Perhaps the act of murder is such an image, the sudden flash of recognition which passes from the patient to us in a moment of extreme conflict. However, this is also the moment of its passing, unsustainable in the aggression which has produced it (Prenelle 2006).

History is not revealed by the momentous events but by the ones that lie hidden in their shadows. This is what brings alive the past in the present, shifting the lens from the subject of history to the history of the subject. Telling stories can be an important source of meaning for patients. Their exploration offers opportunities for individuals with experiences of psychosis to reclaim a sense of their own identity and biography and to escape, at least to some extent, the one-dimensional narratives of pathology. Thus psychotherapy offers such a setting where stories can be told, heard and histories understood. The continuous construction of the meaning of what goes on between patient and analyst reconstructs, in the transference, something of the history of the patient's relationship to his objects, the anxieties involved and the way the defences were built up. The work of reconstruction in analysis is a continuous interweaving of the threads of history, as experienced in the analysis, together with the threads of remembered history, and this combination enriches the patient's understanding of himself, thus providing him with a new autobiography (Riesenberg-Malcolm 1999).

Before murderous acts are committed an inter-psychic boundary crossing occurs, through the use of projective identification. In normal usage, projective identification takes place when an unwanted part of the personality is projected into the other, and then the other, in part-object form, is experienced as if it were the projected content. Klein first named this concept in 1946. In later explorations of the subject, Bion (1959, 1962a, b) did much to differentiate abnormal and normal uses of projective identification, mainly through distinguishing two separate uses: first, as a means of violent evacuation of unwanted parts of the self into the other; and second, as a means of communicating unbearable states of mind. Bion saw the former as a psychotic use of projective identification, which he linked to schizophrenic disturbances due to the level of violence employed, the quality of omnipotent control, the impoverishment to the ego, and the destruction of internal reality. Murderous rage makes use of projective identification to rid the self of intolerable affects which cannot be processed or integrated into the rest of the personality. The violent force of the evacuation in this instance is equivalent to the perceived annihilation to the integrity of the self. This kind of use of projective identification has a paranoid core, which manifests in two different ways: first as a projection of badness, and secondly as a projection of goodness, which we will outline further below. What may be common to both sets of offenders is an underlying vulnerability to shame and exposure.

Projection of badness

In borderline patients, a split between good and bad, between the idealised and the denigrated, in both the inner as well as the external world occurs. In paranoid projective identification, the projection is of badness as seen in paranoid patients. All the hatred and badness is projected outside the self and the individual remains identified with an idealised sense of self which is fragile and weakened by the paranoid phantasies of retaliation and retribution. Klein (1946, p.23) states, 'By introjecting and re-introjecting the forcefully entered object, the subject's feelings of inner persecution are strongly reinforced; all the more since the re-introjected object is felt to contain the dangerous aspects of the self.' In this case the offender attempts to maintain psychic equilibrium by locating danger and badness in others. When the perceived threat is great enough, the offender may be compelled to act out as a perceived act of preservation, or as an attempt to kill off what is threatening to re-enter the self.

The narcissistic exoskeleton – projection of goodness

In the second scenario, the self identifies with idealised people who are held psychically 'outside' so as to keep them away from the buried badness inside (Cartwright 2002). As the narcissistic exoskeleton structure rigidly separating internalised encapsulated badness and externalised goodness becomes less effective or broken down, the patient becomes aware of aspects of himself he cannot tolerate, such as neediness and rage, and so suffers the loss of his idealised version of himself. And because of the long-standing rigid splitting, he has developed little capacity to integrate these aspects of himself. Thus he experiences them psychotically as coming from outside the self, as persecutory attacks. The sequence of the killing begins with weakening of the narcissistic exoskeleton and is followed by its complete collapse, provoked by some particular trigger. The collapse of the defensive structure involves a shift towards identification with a previously buried intolerably bad version of the self. This latter is experienced as an unbearable intrusion which threatens survival. In that moment the threat is evacuated and projected into the victim, who is then experienced as life threatening. The collapse of the narcissistic exoskeleton brings about a violation of boundaries in two ways: first at an intra-psychic level the victim-to-be is a key object in the offender's defensive system. The defensive system cannot function without the victim's compliance in mirroring the existence of the ideal self. When the victim-to-be breaks with his perceived role, this confirms the collapse of the narcissistic exoskeleton. Secondly, all that had been kept at bay now swiftly engulfs the offender, and the boundary between the self and what has been projected collapses.

Cartwright (2002) makes the point that the murderous event usually begins long before the actual attack with the persistent challenging of the defensive organisation, and this may be true in both types of projective identification. Furthermore, the offender is often unable to articulate or represent their levels of distress, due to the nature of the defensive organisation, part of which functions in order to deny or defend against awareness of such difficulties. The build-up to the murderous act then erodes both the offender's attempts at denial as well as the weakening defensive structure. Therefore, along with the weakening of defences, the boundaries between self and other, internal and external, begin to diminish, and at the same time the ever present threat and anxiety increases.

In both scenarios of projective identification, the final murderous attack represents an attempt to destroy the threat, an attempt to annihilate the bad object, at that point experienced concretely within the victim. But not only in the victim; the offender sees the victim as forcing back into them an identification with a bad object which threatens to annihilate their very core. The 'ideal' self is destroyed; there is a forced identification with a persecuted object. In both cases the act of murder is an attempt to create a kind of psychic equilibrium. The fate of the object is less significant in preservative forms of violence. Emphasis is on survival of the self (Glasser 1979). However, this may not happen immediately; it is not always the case that the offender experiences relief in the aftermath of the attack. Usually the offender continues to be haunted and traumatised by his or her actions for some time afterwards. In the aftermath of the murder he or she is forced to confront a disowned part of him- or herself, that is, until his or her narcissistic defences are eventually restored. The defensive organisation then returns with even greater rigidity, often resembling a kind of manic reparation as a wish to reinstate good in their objects. This reinstatement of the defensive organisation, based on encapsulation and projective identification, leads to particular treatment difficulties in working with the homicidal patient, which we will now consider below.

RE-ENACTMENTS WITHIN
THERAPEUTIC RELATIONSHIPS

A difficulty in working with patients who have attained a fragile sense of psychic equilibrium in this way is that the clinician may be left with the challenge, not of working with a volatile, violent patient, but rather of working with 'the model patient' where all the violence and disturbance is evacuated and split off. A large difficulty in psychotherapeutic treatment can be the counter-transference feelings of passivity and boredom as a result of the patient's over-controlling defences. These are patients who can also create enormous 'blind spots' in teams, where there is the danger that the act of murder is overly rationalised, or seen to be a singular historic event, created by a particular set of circumstances and not likely to recur. In this way the real history of the patient is ignored. Staff may be put under enormous pressure to accept the patient's view that they were ill at the time and safe now, stabilised on medication and ready for discharge. Added to this is the pressure to move patients as quickly as possible through the forensic inpatient service and it may be difficult to recognise the real danger, risk and vulnerability these patients present.

Underneath the very calm exterior of the patient, there is often a level of concreteness that demonstrates an ongoing, psychotic, paranoid state where any alternative views are experienced as murderous attacks, which have to be defended against. It can feel persecuting to the patient to continue a line of questioning that differs from their own version of reality. The creation of this rigid structure can stop creative or independent thought in the minds of staff, creating a kind of murder zone that destroys anything that might allow patients to move on and progress. A feature of treatment is how moments of deadlock are reached, where attempts to wonder about links and connections are met with very flat concrete responses, which have the effect of killing meaning. Patients in this scenario could be said to have attempted to get rid of a very dangerous, disturbing part of themselves in the murderous act, and with it the knowledge of their own murderousness. What emerges in the course of this kind of work is how these patients empty themselves out of anything, any feelings, in the act of violently splitting off parts of themselves into others.

Another difficulty is in the encapsulated nature of the offence and the way in which this level of encapsulation is a core aspect of the offender's personality and the way in which their defensive organisation is structured. Due to the over-controlling nature of the personality, symptoms of distress are usually masked and overt signs of psychopathology are often absent. This is another factor which may create blind spots in the treatment team, where similarly the dangerousness of the patient is encapsulated and remains split off. A further extension of this may be where the patient, in resorting to the narcissistic exoskeleton, even elicits the kind of admiration based on a false 'ideal' self. An issue for risk would be a situation where the patient perceives a withdrawal of admiration, leading to a re-enactment of the offence.

WORKING WITH THE HOMICIDAL PATIENT

A large task of the work remains in seeing whether it is possible to arrive at some kind of understanding of the murderous act where some of the patient's projections can be safely withdrawn, in a contained setting, as this is very much linked to levels of insight and also future risk management. However, this is no easy task and it may take many years for this work to begin, if ever. Without this, one may need to see patients as being entirely dependent on a structure in which they can safely be held and contained, and in fact the hospital inpatient setting seems to provide such a structure. We are not suggesting that patients should therefore be indefinitely detained, but careful thought needs to be given to the boundary between inpatient and community settings, and what the crossing of this boundary may mean to patients. The patient is likely to leave not only the security of the hospital environment but also the opportunities for the projection and safe containment of what cannot be borne intra-psychically. Otherwise discharge from the setting may feel like a further boundary violation, an attack on the fragile border between inside and outside.

A treatment goal for these patients may be where there is evidence that there is some possibility for a stronger integration between what is felt to be inside and what has to be kept outside. Once this boundary can begin to be safely crossed and navigated then there is more hope that a patient may be able to manage their own insides, their own anxieties. A salient question on considering discharge may be how safely patients can manage their own anxieties, or whether they will continue to resort to projecting all the anxiety into treatment teams, while they remain 'convinced' they are safe; or alternatively creating a collusive blindness where the temptation is to deny or minimise the level of risk involved. The challenge for treatment teams is how to contain the level of anxiety we are made to feel, both in not acting on it by a wish for patients to be detained indefinitely, and not wishing to get rid of it either by denying the very real risk patients pose to themselves and the public.

REFERENCES

Benjamin, W. (1940) *Theses on the Philosophy of History*. Selected Writing IX.

Bion, W.R. (1959) 'Attacks on Linking.' In *Second Thoughts*. London: Karnac Books (1984).

Bion, W.R. (1962a) 'A Theory of Thinking.' In *Second Thoughts*. London: Karnac Books (1984).

Bion, W.R. (1962b) *Learning from Experience*. Maresfield Reprints. London: Karnac Books (1984).

Cartwright, D. (2002) *Psychoanalysis, Violence and Rage-Type Murder: Murdering Minds*. Hove and New York: Brunner-Routledge.

Doctor, R. (2008) 'A History of Murder.' In Doctor, R. (ed.) *Murder: A Psychotherapeutic Investigation*. Karnac: London.

Glasser, M. (1979) 'Role of aggression in the perversions.' In I. Rosen (ed.) *Sexual Deviation*. Oxford: Oxford Medical Publications.

Klein, M. (1946) 'Notes on Some Schizoid Mechanisms.' In *The Writings of Melanie Klein*. Vol. 3, 1–24.

Prenelle, I. (2006) 'Memory, Modernity and Urban Psychosis.' In M. Heinze *et al.* (eds) *Utopie Heimat*. Berlin: Parados Verlag.

Riesenberg-Malcolm, R. (1999) 'Construction as reliving history.' In *On Bearing Unbearable States of Mind*. London and New York: Routledge.

CONTRIBUTORS

John Adlam is Consultant Adult Psychotherapist in Reflective Practice and Team Development for forensic secure services in South London and Maudsley Foundation NHS Trust and he is also Principal Adult Psychotherapist and Lead for Group Psychotherapies at the South West London and St George's Adult Eating Disorders Service. He trained in Psychoanalytical Group Psychotherapy at the Tavistock Centre and in Forensic Psychotherapeutic Studies at the Portman Clinic. He is a member of the Psycho-Social Studies Network Steering Group and an Associate Editor of the journal *Free Associations*.

Gwen Adshead is a Forensic Psychiatrist and Psychotherapist. She trained at St George's Hospital, the Institute of Psychiatry and the Institute of Group Analysis. She also has a research interest in attachment theory applied to forensic psychiatric services. She has been a consultant forensic psychotherapist for over ten years, at Broadmoor Hospital where she runs therapy groups for offenders. She is also a regular teacher, lecturer and writer: she has written over 100 papers and book chapters on a variety of topics, including forensic psychotherapy, attachment theory and ethics in mental health. She is currently training as a mindfulness teacher; and working on a book about evil. She is also currently President of the International Association for Forensic Psychotherapy.

Anne Aiyegbusi is Deputy Director of Nursing, Specialist and Forensic Services, West London Mental Health NHS Trust. Anne has worked for many years in forensic mental health nursing in the range of registered nursing roles and grades, including that of consultant nurse for women's secure services. Anne has worked across the range of secure mental health settings, including in two high secure hospitals. Her main clinical interest is in integrating attachment theory principles into forensic mental health nursing. Anne is also interested in the manifestation of early traumatic experience in the lives of service users, and in particular, how this reverberates throughout the care system.

Anne has completed a PhD. Her research focused on the nurse-patient relationship with people diagnosed with personality disorders in therapeutic community and secure mental health settings. She has published and made many conference presentations about the psychodynamics of forensic mental health nursing. She has co-edited a book entitled *Therapeutic Relationships with Offenders: An Introduction to the Psychodynamics of Forensic Mental Health Nursing* and is currently the secretary for the International Association for Forensic Psychotherapy.

Andy Benn has worked as a psychologist in high security treatment for 20 years, participating as a therapist in an early intervention RCT for people with a diagnosis of schizophrenia. He has a career-long interest in psychological approaches to working with psychosis and offending. He is currently a Consultant Clinical Psychologist, Chartered Forensic Psychologist, and HPC Registered Clinical and Forensic Psychologist in the Mental Health and National Learning Disability Directorate at Rampton Hospital.

Jo Bownas is consultant systemic family therapist in West London Mental Health NHS Trust, where she works with both adults and adolescents in the London forensic service. She is also a trainer and supervisor of systemic psychotherapists.

Tom Clarke is Associate Director of Nursing South West London and St George's Mental Health NHS Trust and honorary lecturer at Kingston University. Tom is the developer and CEO of POET Health Ltd, an integrated approach to the functional design evaluation of inpatient environments.

Jonathan Coe is the Managing Director of the Clinic for Boundaries Studies, where he has developed new services for professionals. Previously he was CEO of the charity WITNESS(POPAN). In 2009 he completed a Winston Churchill Trust travelling fellowship study tour to the USA, where he visited a wide range of organisations involved in work around professional boundary violations. He acted as a lay member of the Expert Advisory Group for the National Operating Standards for psychological therapies, the Department of Health working group on the Statutory Regulation of Herbal Medicine, Acupuncture and Traditional Chinese Medicine, the Health Professions Council's Professional Liaison Groups for Counselling and Psychology and the Ethics Committee of the British Psychological Society. He was a member of the steering group for the Council for Healthcare Regulatory Excellence's Clear Sexual Boundaries Project. He has worked in mental health services for the last 25 years.

Richard Curen has worked as a psychotherapist, counsellor and manager in the sexual abuse field for the last 17 years. Until recently he was Chief Executive and is currently the Consultant Forensic Psychotherapist at Respond. Previously he worked at Survivors UK, where, amongst other things, he was responsible for managing the individual and group psychotherapy services for adult male survivors of sexual violence. Richard has also worked as a group facilitator at the Domestic Violence Intervention Project and as a men's counsellor at Orexis – a community drug project in South East London. He is a board member of both the International Association for Forensic Psychotherapy and the Institute of Psychotherapy and Disability. Richard is also a member of the National Association for the Treatment of Abusers, a member of the Tavistock Society of Psychotherapists and Allied Professionals and a visiting Lecturer at the Tavistock and Portman NHS Trust.

Brian Darnley is a Consultant Psychiatrist in Forensic Psychotherapy working for Devon Partnership NHS Trust. He runs an inpatient unit for severely personality disordered women and is currently involved in developing pathways of care for personality disordered offenders.

Stella Compton Dickinson has worked in forensic services for over fifteen years. Whilst employed as Clinical Research Lead in Arts Therapies at Rampton hospital (UK) for over ten years, she has presented and published developments internationally; manualised and implemented research trials in forensic music therapy; and contributed to and edited a book on Forensic Music Therapy (Jessica Kingsley Publishers). Stella is an Honorary Research Fellow at the Institute of Mental Health, Nottingham, a fellow of the Royal Society of Arts, and holds an Honorary Research Contract at the Institute of Psychiatry, Health Service and Population Research Department.

Dawn Devereux is Director of Public Support at the Clinic for Boundaries Studies and a psychotherapist in private practice. She has a PhD in ethics and Psychotherapy and publishes and researches on the subject.

Claire Dimond is an Adolescent Forensic Psychiatrist. She has worked as a consultant in a community CAMHS, Feltham YOI and the Wells unit. The Wells unit is a secure adolescent forensic service for adolescent males.

Ronald Doctor is a Consultant Psychiatrist in Psychotherapy, West London Mental Health NHS Trust. He was Academic Secretary of the Royal College of Psychiatrists Psychotherapy Faculty. He is Chair of the NHS Liaison Committee, British Psychoanalytical Society, Chair of the Association of Psychoanalytical Psychotherapy in the NHS, (APP) and Honorary Clinical Lecturer at Imperial College. He has edited two books: *Dangerous Patients: A Psychodynamic Approach to Risk Assessment and Management* and *Murder: A Psychotherapeutic Investigation*.

Glen Gabbard earned his Bachelor's Degree in Theatre from Eastern Illinois University and an MD from Rush Medical College in Chicago in 1975. He completed his psychiatry residency at the Karl Menninger School of Psychiatry in Topeka, Kansas. He then served on the staff of the Menninger Clinic for 26 years and served as Director of the Menninger Hospital from 1989 to 1994 and Director of the Topeka Institute for Psychoanalysis from 1996 to 2001. He moved to Baylor College of Medicine in 2001. He founded the Gabbard Center in July 2011. Glen has authored or edited 24 books and over 300 papers, including a book on media depictions of psychiatry and mental illness in films with his brother Krin. He was Joint Editor-in-Chief of the *International Journal of Psychoanalysis* and was Associate Editor of the *American Journal of Psychiatry*. Awards include the Strecker Award for outstanding psychiatrist under age 50 in 1994, the Sigourney Award for Outstanding Contributions to Psychoanalysis in 2000, the American Psychiatric Association Distinguished Service Award in 2002, the American Psychiatric Association Adolf Meyer Award in 2004, and the Rush Medical College Distinguished Alumnus in 2005.

Mario Guarnieri is a Psychoanalytic Psychotherapist and Dramatherapist. Between 1999 and 2009 he worked at both Broadmoor High Secure Hospital and Three Bridges Medium Secure Hospital, West London Mental Health NHS Trust. Currently, he is working at Croydon Personality Disorder Service based at Bethlem Royal Hospital, South London and Maudsley NHS Foundation Trust. Mario has contributed to a number of presentations and publications about his work. He also has a private practice and a freelance practice which includes consultancy work with Broadmoor Hospital multi-disciplinary staff teams.

David Jones is a psychoanalytic psychotherapist. He has worked in Her Majesty's Prison Service, at the therapeutic prison HMP Grendon and as Consultant Psychotherapist in Forensic Psychiatry at Millfields, a medium secure unit developed as part of the Dangerous and Severe Personality Disorder (DSPD) project. Currently he is an independent consultant in group and institutional dynamics and Expert Therapeutic Community Adviser to the Royal College of Psychiatry, Community of Communities, a quality network of therapeutic communities.

He is the editor of two books, *Working with Dangerous People* and *Humane Prisons*, and has published a number of papers focusing on the psychopathology of offenders and the difficulties faced by institutions, particularly institutions in the public sector, including the National Health Service and the prison service.

Gillian Kelly (Nee Tuck) is a Consultant Nurse at West London Mental Health Trust. She has worked in medium and high secure mental health services for the last 10 years, specialising in the care of patients who have personality disorder. She has particular interests in working with women in secure care, the psychodynamics of forensic mental health nursing and the use of a systems-psychodynamic approach to examining organisations. Gillian led the development of a Boundaries Workshop and has several years' experience in facilitating boundaries training across all disciplines. Gillian has completed a Master's Degree in *Consultation and the Organisation: Psychoanalytic Approaches* at the Tavistock Centre.

Gabriel Kirtchuk is a Consultant Psychiatrist in Psychotherapy and a Psychoanalyst. He has worked in forensic settings for the last seventeen years and has established a Department of Forensic Psychotherapy, at the Three Bridges, West London Mental Health NHS Trust. He is also the Lead Clinician of the National Forensic Psychotherapy Training and Development Strategy, as well as the Chair of the Special Interest Group in Forensic Psychotherapy at the Royal College of Psychiatrists. He is an honorary clinical senior lecturer at Imperial College London and is a fellow of the British Psychoanalytical Society. His areas of interest have been the development of psychotherapeutic approaches within forensic mental health as well as training and educational programmes in this field.

Stephen Mackie is a Consultant Forensic Nurse Psychotherapist at the Portman Clinic, Tavistock and Portman NHS Foundation Trust. He has many years' experience of providing reflective practice consultations to low and medium secure organisations and draws upon this experience in his contribution to the present volume. He is a member of the Lincoln Centre for Psychotherapy and also works in private practice in London.

Maggie McAlister is a Jungian Analyst (SAP) and works as a Highly Specialised Adult Psychotherapist within a Forensic Psychotherapy Dept within the NHS. She previously worked as a Dramatherapist for over fourteen years in general and forensic psychiatry and has published several papers on arts therapies and psychotherapy in the field of adult mental health. She is a Senior Lecturer for the MSc in Psychotherapeutic Approaches to Mental Health jointly run by Bucks New University and West London Mental Health Trust.

Estelle Moore is an HPC registered Clinical and Forensic Psychologist and Chartered Scientist, who has worked in high secure services for more than 15 years. Her current role is the lead for the Centralised Groupwork Service on Newbury Therapy Unit at Broadmoor Hospital, which is a multi-disciplinary service she co-founded over a decade ago, where she operates as a group facilitator and supervisor. Alongside this, she has an active research and clinical interest in building alliances that promote successful outcomes in forensic settings. Estelle is a member of the Forensic Recovery Project Team (supported by the NHS Confederation, Department of Health and Centre for Mental Health), working towards the promotion of recovery in secure settings.

Anna Motz is a Consultant Clinical and Forensic Psychologist and Psychotherapist with extensive clinical experience with women as perpetrators of violence and with the staff teams who work with them. She is currently working in the forensic services at Oxfordhealth Foundation Trust. She is the author of *The Psychology of Female Violence: Crimes Against the Body* (Routledge 2001, 2008), editor of *Managing Self Harm: Psychological Perspectives* (Routledge 2009) and author of the forthcoming book *Toxic Couples: The Psychology of Violent Relationships* (Routledge 2013), and is a past president of The International Association for Forensic Psychotherapy.

Rebecca Neeld was formerly Lead Nurse at the Cassel Hospital 2001–11, and is now a group psychotherapist at the Cassel Hospital, West London Mental Health NHS Trust with special interests in services for people with personality disorders.

Kingsley Norton qualified in medicine at Clare College, Cambridge, thereafter pursuing a career in psychiatry at St George's, London, obtaining his MD (Cantab) in 1988. He qualified as a Jungian Analyst in 1989 (Society of Analytical Psychologists) and has held Consultant appointments in General Psychiatry (1984–89) and in Psychotherapy (Director, Henderson Hospital, 1989–2006) and West London Mental Health Trust (2006 to date). He has written and researched extensively in the fields of Personality Disorder, Therapeutic Communities, and healthcare organisation. He has written/ co-written four books. As PD clinical lead in his current post, he remains committed to improving the service received by people diagnosed with Personality Disorder. He has also been involved in leading the Trust's response to the 'Clear Boundaries' initiative over the last five years.

Derek Perkins is a Consultant Clinical and Forensic Psychologist and Head of Psychological Services at Broadmoor Hospital. He was co-founder of the forensic psychology training course at the University of Surrey, where he is a Visiting Professor of Forensic Psychology. His research interests include sexual offending and personality disorder, and the psychophysiological assessment of offence-related sexual interests. He has published a number of papers and book chapters on forensic psychology and sexual offending, and was recently part of an international forum on sexual homicide and paraphilias, which is published as a book of the same name by the Correctional Service Canada.

Cindy Peternelj-Taylor is a Professor with the College of Nursing, University of Saskatchewan, a Distinguished Fellow with the International Association of Forensic Nurses, and Editor of the *Journal of Forensic Nursing*. Her research and scholarship focuses on professional role development for nurses and other healthcare professionals who work with vulnerable populations in forensic psychiatric and correctional settings, with particular emphasis on ethical issues (e.g. boundary violations, othering) that emerge from practice. Her current research explores the lived experience of nurse engagement with forensic patients in secure environments.

Emma Ramsden is an HPC registered Dramatherapist and Clinical Supervisor who has worked in high secure services for more than 10 years. Alongside this work, she has extensive experience in the fields of addiction, violent behaviour and in educational settings as both therapist and behaviour consultant, with children and families in deprived settings. Emma is in the closing stages of her doctoral research at Leeds Metropolitan University, where she has been exploring children's rights to consent as co-researchers in their own therapeutic intervention.

David Reiss is a consultant forensic psychiatrist at West London Mental Health NHS Trust, and an honorary clinical senior lecturer at Imperial College London. His research examines the interface between clinical forensic psychiatry and public policy, including work on homicide inquiries, stalking, interpersonal dynamics and educational issues. His clinical and educational work focuses on enabling the multi-disciplinary team to gain an enhanced understanding of patients, thereby improving care and reducing risk. He is the author of numerous journal papers and co-editor of the book *Containment in the Community*.

Christopher Scanlon is Consultant Psychotherapist in general adult and forensic mental health with the lead for group psychotherapy and reflective practice and team development, Department of Psychotherapy, South London and Maudsley Foundation NHS Trust; Training Group Analyst and member of the teaching faculty, Institute of Group Analysis (London); visiting senior lecturer in Forensic Psychotherapy at St George's University of London; Senior Visiting Research Fellow, Centre for Psycho-social Studies, University of West England (UWE); associate member of Organisation for Promotion of the Understanding of Society (OPUS); full member of the International Society for the Psychoanalytic Study of Society (ISPSO); associate editor for

Psychoanalysis, Culture and Society and *Free Associations,* and an Independent
Psychotherapist Educator and Organisational Consultant. He was previously
Consultant Psychotherapist and lead for Training and Consultation at
Henderson Hospital Democratic Therapeutic Community Services;
professional adviser to the Department of Health's Personality Disorder
Expert Advisory Group and the 'Social Inclusion Unit' in the Department
for Communities and Local Government (formerly the Office of the Deputy
Prime Minister), and a trustee of the Zito Trust – a major UK Mental Health
Charity campaigning for improved services for mentally disordered offenders
and their victims.

Denise Sullivan is a mental health nurse. She has worked with young people
in both community and forensic CAMHS. She is currently the lead nurse for
mental health services in the HMYOI Feltham and the Wells Unit.

Emma Wadey is a Consultant Nurse for the Personality Directorate at
Broadmoor High Secure Hospital. Her clinical work focuses on working with
patients with complex trauma and with nursing colleagues to develop, nurture
and sustain a culture of therapeutic engagement supported by the development
of bespoke training packages and the facilitation of clinical supervision and
reflective practice.

SUBJECT INDEX

Sub-headings in *italics* indicate tables and figures.

AUTHOR INDEX